# Health Care UK Autumn 2001

The King's Fund review of health policy

Edited by John Appleby and Anthony Harrison

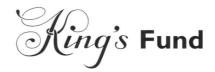

Published by
King's Fund Publishing
11–13 Cavendish Square
London W1G 0AN

© King's Fund 2001

First published 2001

ISBN 1 85717 437 2

A CIP catalogue record for this book is
available from the British Library

Available from:

King's Fund Bookshop
11–13 Cavendish Square
London
W1G 0AN

Tel:    020 7307 2591
Fax:    020 7307 2801

Printed and bound in Great Britain

*Cover image: Minuche Mazumdar Farrar*

# CONTENTS

# POLICY ANALYSIS

# DATASCAN

# CONTRIBUTORS

John Appleby
*Director, Health Systems Programme, King's Fund*

Naaz Coker
*Director, Race and Diversity, King's Fund*

Anna Coote
*Director, Public Health Programme, King's Fund*

Michael Damiani
*Senior Analyst, King's Fund*

Jennifer Dixon
*Director, Health Care Policy Programme, King's Fund*

Teresa Edmans
*Programme Manager, Health and Regeneration, King's Fund*

Angela Greatley
*Fellow in Mental Health, King's Fund*

Anthony Harrison
*Senior Fellow in Health Systems, King's Fund*

Bobbie Jacobson
*Director, London Health Observatory*

Jo-Ann Mulligan
*Research Officer, Health Systems Programme, King's Fund*

Ruth Tennant
*Programme Manager, Imagine London, King's Fund*

Valerie Wildridge
*Enquiry Services Librarian, King's Fund Library*

David Woodhead
*Fellow in Public Health, King's Fund*

# In this issue

*London's Public Health Observatory ... community safety ... London on the Internet ... public attitudes towards the NHS ... mental health in the capital*

## John Appleby

The theme for this issue of HCUK is London, its health and health care services. Around 7 million people live in the capital – 12 per cent of the UK population. Its health services consume £7 billion a year – 6 per cent of London's GDP. As with all large conurbations, London has extremes of poverty and wealth, and illness and health. It also faces some unique challenges in co-ordinating its health care services.

The King's Fund – more fully, the King Edward's Hospital Fund for London – has provided support for London's hospitals since 1897. The introduction of the NHS and other developments has meant that its focus has changed over the last century, but its central mission is to improve the health of Londoners. Through a mixture of grant giving, policy analysis, service development, education, training and other activities, the Fund plays a part in improving health services and the wider health-influencing environment.

This edition reflects some of the Fund's current work relating to London, but starts with an overview of a new development in public health within the NHS – Health Observatories. **Bobbie Jacobson** sets out the thinking behind London's Public Health Observatory (one of eight in England) and its plans for the future. Launched in February 2000, the Observatory will not only provide statistical and information support on health issues to London's NHS, but will also be the lead Observatory on two important issues: health inequalities and regeneration, and social exclusion.

In a year in which there was a general election, it is hard to avoid public opinion polls. During May and early June, newspapers and television reported daily on the results of new polls. For many years, the King's Fund has carried out *ad hoc* surveys of the public to ascertain views about the NHS in general and specific attitudes on particular aspects of health and health care. This year, in conjunction with London's *Evening Standard*, the Fund carried out a pre-election poll of Londoners' attitudes towards the NHS and health issues in general. **Jo-Ann Mulligan** reports on the findings of the poll and, interestingly (for politicians at least), notes the gap between how people would like the NHS to change (or not) and whether they think their preferred change is likely to happen.

Despite a range of new initiatives designed to improve mental health services and greater central guidance, **Angela Greatley** asks whether the NHS will manage to achieve significant change over the coming years – in particular, whether it will be able to improve on a 1997 King's Fund assessment that characterised London's mental health services as containing pockets of good practice barely discernible within a generally gloomy environment.

Within the UK, London is a key destination for asylum seekers and refugees. As **Naaz Coker** writes, such people often face unique health problems arising not only from their traumatic experiences in their home country, but also from social difficulties once in London. Accessing NHS facilities can be difficult for all of us at one time or another, but navigating such a complex system

when you do not speak English, and when you may be feeling culturally and socially disoriented, can be doubly difficult.

Another potentially vulnerable group is children. As **Ruth Tennant** and **Teresa Edmans** point out, London contains some stark disparities in the life chances of children: a child in Tower Hamlets is twice as likely to die before it reaches four than a child in Richmond, for example. The Government's response to such inequalities and growing pressure to tackle child poverty and social exclusion has been a number of fiscal and supply-side initiatives – from Sure Start to New Deals for communities. As the authors note, co-ordinating such a baffling range of developments across government is not going to be easy. Moreover, evaluation of these interventions is proving difficult.

Another area in which evaluation has proved hard is in arriving at an understanding of the way demand for emergency services changes – and, in particular, seasonal variations in demand (whisper it: 'winter crises'). Using data for London

from the Hospital Episode Statistics, **Michael Damiani** and **Jennifer Dixon** describe early findings from their investigation into the highs and lows of emergency demand in London. From weekly reports of emergency admissions, it is clear that respiratory diseases are the key problem for the NHS in winter, affecting the young and the old. The results of this analysis should help the NHS focus on at-risk people to provide, for example, more proactive preventative interventions and so ease pressures during winter.

The history of planning health services and developing pan-London health strategies in the capital could best be summed up as disjointed. With 16 (though decreasing) health authorities, 33 boroughs, 59 trusts, and over 4000 general practitioners, London is a tangle of overlapping organisational boundaries. But in the last few years things have started to change. Now there is just one NHS regional office for London and, importantly, a new authority – the Greater London Authority – and, unique in the UK, an elected mayor charged, in part, with the responsibility to tackle health issues. **Anna Coote** and **Ruth Tennant** tell the story of how these new organisations came into being and how the newly formed London Health Commission is moving towards a proper health strategy for the capital.

The Commission's health strategy will, of course, cast its net widely, taking into account the health impact of policies and actions outside the NHS – transport, regeneration, etc. – but which impact on Londoners' health. One

issue that, as **David Woodhead** notes, many Londoners complain about is crime and the fear of crime. Views about community safety (an umbrella term covering a range of physical and psychological safety issues) emphasise the links with health and also the role that the NHS can and should play together with other agencies and groups to ensure a safer environment for Londoners. Co-ordination, commitment and – yes – money are key to success in this enterprise.

Finally, what could be seen as a useful article published in completely the wrong media. Information about Internet sites printed on paper makes a mockery of the unique contribution the Internet has to offer – clickable hypertext links! Nevertheless, **Valerie Wildridge**'s rough guide to Internet sites devoted to health and health care in London will also be available on the King's Fund web site (www.kingsfund.org.uk).

# The new London Health Observatory: for whose benefit?

## Bobbie Jacobson

In February 2000, the then Minister of State for Public Health, Tessa Jowell, launched England's eight brand new Public Health Observatories (PHOs) – one in each health region. This was part of the Government's response to the White Paper *Saving Lives: Our Healthier Nation*.[1] It is the job of each Observatory to support its local and regional partners to:

- monitor health and disease trends and implications for action
- identify gaps in health information
- advise on methods for health and health inequality impact assessments
- bring together information on health from different sources to support health improvement
- undertake focused work on special topics

- evaluate local progress in tackling health inequalities and improving health
- alert policy-makers and stakeholders to future public health problems.

The recently announced changes in the regional tier of the NHS and the development of devolved government mean that the Observatories have an important role to play in contributing to an integrated public health function in each region, and in ensuring that the health voice is heard across regional government.

### CREATING NATIONAL AND REGIONAL PARTNERSHIPS

While working primarily to serve health priorities within each of the eight regions, the PHOs also work as a national network – the Association of Public Health Observatories

(APHO). This enables us to put cross-regional expertise together to help tackle some common problems, such as access to common core data needed in every region. The APHO has undertaken a number of national projects for the Department of Health and others, and will be publishing its first annual review in July,[2] together with a new report reviewing the methodological issues we need to tackle to obtain useful public health information at PCG/T level.[3]

Each Observatory has been designated a lead or link Observatory in a number of key health and health care policy areas. The London Health Observatory (LHO) is the link for two areas: health inequalities and regeneration, and social exclusion.

## THE LONDON HEALTH OBSERVATORY

The LHO is unique in many important respects. First, and most important, it serves by far the largest and mostly richly diverse regions in the country. Second, it has been established at a time of unprecedented change in London's governance. It is the first region in England with an elected mayor and devolved regional government, in which not only are geographical boundaries shared, but improving health and tackling inequalities is a goal shared by Mayor Ken Livingstone, the Greater London Authority (GLA) *and* the London Office of the NHSE. An indication of the strength of that shared partnership comes from the integrated public health leadership provided by London's Regional Director of Public Health for the NHS (also the mayor's health adviser).

The LHO is also unique in that it encompasses England's largest concentration of health research and intelligence capacity, distributed across a myriad of complex university, local statutory and non-statutory partners.

About 70 per cent of London's NHS R&D resources come to London. To maximise the outputs of such a treasury would need the invention of the LHO if it didn't already exist. In the highly competitive R&D climate, one of the important tasks for the LHO will be to create and support networks of participating partners.

## WHO RUNS THE LHO?

Stakeholder consultation led to the view that the LHO needed to be developed with the capacity to be a source of credible health intelligence, working with key partners, but not being subsumed by any. This will enable the LHO to work with and raise resources from a wide range of sponsors. As a result, the LHO will be led by an independently appointed chair and a multi-agency management board drawn from both pan-London and local interests. The LHO is a member of the London Health Commission, which acts as a stakeholder reference group for the LHO.

The LHO has offices at the King's Fund, which it shares with the Health of Londoners Programme (HOLP) – a key programme within the LHO.

## WHAT CAN THE LHO DO FOR USERS?

The LHO is still at an early stage of development. Its ideas are big, but its objectives must be achievable. The LHO has a well-developed web site (www.lho.org.uk) that provides health information and data, and signposts users to other sources of information they might need on health in London. Keeping an overview of the changing sea of health web sites is an important network function for London's health. This is essential to help 'signpost' users to appropriate sources of health intelligence and to avoid time-wasting and duplication of effort. Our analysis of web site use so far has shown that users from the private sector and across Europe featured nearly as significantly as NHS and local government partners. We expect that NHS and local partners across London will make much more use of the web site over time once they know what is on offer.

But the LHO is also committed to developing a responsive health intelligence function that is more than simply a web site. To widen and deepen access to health intelligence we will be developing a 'query desk' to complement our web site work. We hope this 'human signpost' will help less confident users – perhaps in local authorities, primary care and the voluntary sector – to access relevant information on the health of Londoners. We will develop a system for prioritising information requests and will work with the voluntary sector and others to develop a user group to help lead this work.

## SUPPORTING THE STRATEGIC AGENDA FOR HEALTH IN LONDON

The LHO is committed to supporting the London Health Strategy,[4] now widely agreed across pan-London and local agencies and led by the London Health Commission (LHC). The LHC was established by the London Regional Office working with the mayor and GLA (see www.londonshealth.gov.uk). The London Health Strategy has four overarching priorities:

- regeneration and health
- black and ethnic minority health
- tackling inequalities in health
- transport and health.

LHO and its partner health intelligence programme, HOLP, have already contributed to each of these priorities, with further work underway.[5] Key pieces of work in progress within LHO and HOLP include:

- mapping the new national inequalities targets and projecting them for London, and supporting the development of local action plans
- assessing the burden of illness and costs of road accidents to Londoners and London's services
- supporting the development and audit of the highest standards of prevention, treatment and care for families affected by sickle cell disease and haemoglobin-related disorders
- developing a black and ethnic health monitoring/intelligence function to plug gaps in what we know
- developing a *Guide to Planning in Health and Local Authorities* for the 'uninitiated'
- developing a toolbox of indicators to help monitor the health effects of regeneration programmes.

## DEVELOPING PUBLIC HEALTH CAPACITY IN LONDON

At a time when NHS organisations are changing rapidly, it is vital to ensure that the public health function thrives at all levels in the system – from government through to regions and local health economies.[6] The creation of PCTs and the Local Strategic Partnership means that the demand for specialist expertise will increase not decrease. The LHO intends to play a significant support role, not only in supporting multidisciplinary trainees in public health, but also in developing a London-wide training programme and network to enable practitioners in local government, NHS and the voluntary sector to develop basic and more advanced skills needed for local health impact assessment work.

This work is already well embedded in all nine of the mayor's health strategies. The LHO is currently working with the GLA to provide the evidence base to support the HIA for the mayor's London Plan. We want the health impact assessment training programme to result not only in better health-orientated policy-making and practice in London, but also to create a much needed increase in public health capacity and awareness in London's local organisations.

## REFERENCES

1 Department of Health. *Saving lives: our healthier nation*. London: HMSO, 1999.

2 Association of Public Health Observatories. *www.pho.org.uk*

3 Bardsley M *et al. Developing public health information for PCGs/Ts. Methodological issues*. In press.

4 Coalition for Health and Regeneration. *The London health strategy*. Also available at *www.londonshealth.gov.uk*

5 London Health Observatory. *LHO briefing No. 1*. May 2001.

6 CMO report of the Public Health Function, February 1998. *www.doh.gov.uk/cmo/cmoproj.htm*

# Key events in health care

Anthony Harrison

## OVERVIEW

As we recorded in the Winter 2000 edition of *Health Care UK*, by early 2000 the Government had succeeded in meeting its election commitment to reduce waiting lists for hospital treatment to 100,000 below the figure it inherited. That achievement had been maintained in the period running up to the election.

The form of this target – its focus on numbers waiting rather than waiting times – had been the object of criticism ever since its publication. The NHS Plan indicated that this point had been addressed by setting targets for improved access in terms of maximum waiting times. Furthermore, it also acknowledged that to reduce waiting times there had to be a higher level of activity. During the election campaign, the Secretary of State made that explicit by setting out in precise terms the number of extra operations it was intended to bring about. In a speech on 24 May, he said that by 2005 there would be 140,000 more hip, hernia, knee and cataract operations, an increase of some 35 per cent over the current figure.

During the four months covered in this edition of *Health Care UK*, the Government provided plenty of evidence of its determination to press ahead with implementing the proposals set out in the Plan. The entries below record the Government's plans for increasing the number of professional staff in training, including the establishment of two new medical schools and other measures such as changes to the consultant contract, new payments to GPs and dentists to encourage staff retention, and the construction of new hospitals and other facilities.

In addition, the national service framework for older people and a new strategy – a national service framework in all but name – for those with learning disabilities were published, and a new National Cancer Institute was set up – a direct response to the critical report published last year from the House of Commons Science and Technology Committee. All these measures embody strong central direction.

The Secretary of State's speech on 25 April 2001 was therefore all the more surprising. Not only did it appear to represent an about-turn – back, in fact, to the 1997 White Paper – but it also indicated that structural changes, which the 1997 White Paper had suggested would be kept to a minimum, were far from over. The abolition of regional offices and the reduction in the number of health authorities to around 30 could be, and indeed was, a step towards allowing localities to 'get on with the job'. But the job itself – meeting the targets set out in the Plan and in subsequent statements – remains centrally defined.

While the Plan and its implementation provided the main business of the four months, there were other developments of note, for example, the report on climate change and the proposals to expand genetic services (together with the Science and Technology Select Committee report, *Genetics and Insurance*, published in April 2001).

The Calendar also notes a number of public health measures. In contrast to those bearing on the reform of services, they appear modest and tentative. In March, the House of Commons Health Committee published a review of how the Government's public health policies were working. Its report concluded that 'a great opportunity to give public health a real impetus has been lost by the lack of emphasis in this area in the Plan'. Because of the election, the Government did not publish a formal reply during the period covered by this review.

## FEBRUARY

2  **Cardiac care:** £3.7 million announced for purchase of cardiac equipment.

7  **Research and development:** budget for research and development increased by 6.6. per cent to £479 million:

> The NHS Research & Development budget will be £479 million in 2001/02, an increase of 6.6 per cent on 2000/01. The funding provides more than £20 million for new research and development to take forward the NHS Plan, including research in cancer, coronary heart disease and mental health, and health technology assessments for the National Institute for Clinical Excellence. (Press release 2001/0169, p.1)

**Health authority budgets:** an extra £140 million allocated to health authorities, bringing the total average increase for 2001/02 to 8.9 per cent.

8  **NHS Direct:** following the recommendations made in the Independent Review of GP Out-of-Hours Services, measures were announced to implement proposed unification of NHS Direct and GP co-operatives at local level.

**Child poverty:** £60 million allocated to reducing child poverty in low-income areas, to be used to extend Sure Start programme to include pregnant women and their partners for the first time.

9  **Climate:** Department of Health published comprehensive report on the effects of climate change. The report predicts:

- cold-related winter deaths are likely to decrease substantially, by perhaps 20,000 per annum

- heat-related summer deaths are likely to increase, by around 2800 cases per annum
- cases of food poisoning are likely to increase significantly, by perhaps 10,000 cases per annum
- insect-borne diseases may present local problems, but the increase in their overall impact is likely to be small
- water-borne diseases may increase, but the overall impact is likely to be small
- the risk from disasters caused by severe winter gales and coastal flooding is likely to increase
- in general, the effects of air pollutants on health are likely to decline, but the effects of ozone during the summer are likely to increase; several thousand extra deaths and a similar number of hospitals admissions may occur each year
- cases of skin cancer are likely to increase by up to 5000 cases per year and cataracts by 2000 cases per year
- measures taken to reduce the rate of climate change by reducing greenhouse gas emissions could produce secondary beneficial effects on health. (Press release 2001/0074, pp.1–2)

**Maternity care:** working group on maternity services established to find the best way of providing services that provide safe, effective, evidence-based and accessible care.

12 **Drug misuse:** £25 million allocated for a programme to:

- expand and provide new treatment services
- increase the numbers of misusers in treatment programmes

- train and recruit drug counsellors, and provide training for drugs and mental health workers in dual diagnosis
- improve training and raise awareness amongst doctors and nurses about drugs
- achieve more supervised 'ingestion of methadone' schemes, and reduce injecting drug use and sharing of needles to prevent blood-borne diseases.

Over £12 million of the additional funding has been given directly to health authorities in order to:

- improve access and increase availability of treatment services for drug misusers
- support initiatives to reduce drug-related deaths, diversion of prescription drugs, injecting drug use and sharing of needles.

Extra cash will also be focused on the main themes of drug education, prevention programmes, training and counselling. Around 8000 health practitioners, including GPs, nurses and pharmacists, will receive training in drug misuse to improve their skills and expertise. (Press release 2001/0076, p.1)

**Nursing:** new nurses recruitment campaign launched, focused on encouraging trained nurses, midwives and other health professionals to return to the NHS.

**Dentistry:** new dentistry commitment scheme introduced, which will involve:

- an increased number of steps in the scheme to ensure dentists' commitment to the NHS is better recognised

- better recognition of commitment shown by dentists accepting treatment on referral
- the minimum earnings for qualification for the main scheme being lowered from £50,000 to £40,000
- recognition of other important NHS activity that dentists undertake, for example supporting training and working with health authorities to improve oral health. (Press release 2001/0083, p.1)

**15 Service planning:** Health Service Circular (HSC 2001/03) *Implementing the NHS Plan: Developing Services Following the National Beds Inquiry*, requires each health authority, along with councils and other partners, to:

- examine the information about their current pattern of use of services, relative to other areas, as evidenced by the updated analysis (paragraphs 14–15)
- consider what changes will be needed to make their contribution to the NHS Plan's objectives for 7000 additional beds by 2004 (paragraphs 16–18). At present, no health authority should plan for a reduction in beds, including general and acute beds, unless there is very clear justification based on exceptional local circumstances. Where this is the case, the plans will need to be endorsed explicitly by the appropriate Regional Office, in consultation with the Department of Health head-quarters. The priority must be to ensure that sufficient capacity exists to expand services, enhance the quality of services and meet agreed targets

- feed this analysis into their local performance and modernisation audit, and submit their proposals, signed off by all partners, to the appropriate NHS and Social Care Regional Offices, indicating what proposals are intended to be included in the 2001–02 HIMP. (p.3)

**Staffing:** increase in training budgets announced for doctors, nurses and other staff. This will mean that:

- between now and 2009, the numbers of consultants will rise from 24,300 to 36,300 – an increase of at least 12,000 (49%) – with significant rises in the priority areas of CHD and cancer. Over the next ten years we expect cancer consultant numbers to increase by 55% and CHD consultant numbers to increase by 83%
- between 2000 and 2009, the numbers of midwives is set to rise from 22,600 to 32,600 – an increase of at least 10,000 (44%)
- between 2000 and 2009, the numbers of nurses and midwives is set to rise from 343,000 to 403,200 – an increase of at least 59,600 (17%)
- between 2000 and 2009, the numbers of physiotherapists is set to rise from 15,600 to 24,800 – an increase of at least 9,200 (59%)
- between 2000 and 2009, the numbers of GPs is set to rise from 28,600 to 31,600 – an increase of 3000 (10%). (Press release 2001/0087, p.1)

**Hospitals:** 29 hospital schemes announced, costing £3.1 million. Sixteen will include 'fast track' treatment centres. A further ten such centres were also announced.

**21 Consultants:** proposals announced for new consultant pay scales in return for doing less private practice:

- the proposals could mean the average consultant earning £82,500 ten years after being appointed – almost £20,000 more than under the current arrangements
- more consultants would also be eligible for access to an expanded new clinical awards scheme to replace the outdated 'merit' awards on top of their basic pay
- under the proposals, newly qualified consultants would need to work exclusively for the NHS for a period of perhaps seven years. There would also be better planning and clearer specifications throughout consultants' careers of what the NHS expects from them
- current consultants – as well as newly appointed consultants – could also be eligible for these new benefits if they meet the new criteria. (Press release 2001/0092, p.1)

**22 Nursing:** new nursing standards set out in *The Essence of Care*, covering:

- principles of self-care
- personal and oral hygiene
- nutrition
- continence and bladder and bowel care
- pressure ulcers
- safety with clients with mental health needs
- record keeping
- privacy and dignity. (Press release 2001/0096, p.2)

**27 Organ donations:** targets announced to:

- double the number of people on the organ donation register from 8 million to 16 million by 2010
- develop a national service framework (NSF) for patients with kidney failure to establish national standards and improve services
- increase the kidney transplant rate by almost 100% by 2005
- increase heart, lung and liver transplants by 10% by 2005
- establish a new national consultative body to consider and offer advice on all transplant issues. (Press release 2001/0104, p.1)

**28 Diet:** pilots of the National Schools Fruit Scheme announced, covering 500 schools, most in Health Action Zones.

**Smoking:** Government welcomed new EU agreement on tobacco advertising. The draft text states that the directive:

… strengthens health warnings on tobacco products to include references to passive smoking, ageing of the skin and impotence caused by smoking. Misleading descriptors which suggest that some tobacco products are safer than others will be banned in future. (Press release 2001/0109, p.1)

**Health inequalities:** the first health inequalities targets announced:

The new infant mortality target aims to reduce the gap in infant deaths between different social classes. Starting with children under one year, the target for 2010 will be to reduce by at least 10 per cent the gap in infant mortality rates between manual groups and the population as a whole. There is also a target to reduce by at least 10 per cent the gap between the fifth of health authorities with the lowest life expectancy at birth and the population as a whole by 2010. (Press release 2001/0108, p.1)

**Health professionals:** *Making the Change* published, a strategy for improving the training and career opportunities for health care scientists working in the NHS. It provides for:

- a new career structure for health care scientists to replace the outdated national grades, more opportunities to combine or move between jobs in practice, education and research, and better rewards for working in expanded roles
- a commitment to modernise and reshape education and training pathways so that staff receive the highest-quality training and ongoing development
- a commitment to develop more flexible career pathways so that high-quality staff can be recruited and retrained
- a major project to develop a national occupational standards framework to enhance public confidence
- a review of the health care scientist workforce to ensure adequate numbers of professional staff are available to deliver high-quality scientific services
- extension of 'NHS Careers', a multi-media careers service, to cover the health care science workforce. (Press release 2001/0107)

## MARCH

1 **Heart surgery:** £60 million announced for the expansion and improvement of heart surgery services, particularly in areas with high levels of heart disease.

**Research and development:** a new framework published for the governance of health and social care research.

5 **NHS Direct:** results of caller satisfaction survey over Christmas 2000 found that:

- 96% of callers are either satisfied or very satisfied with the service
- 97% of respondents said that they got through the first time they called. 2% got through on their second attempt
- 96% of respondents described the advice they were given as helpful and 100% of those that answered said they were clear about what the nurse was advising they should do next
- 68% of callers said that they would either call NHS Direct again or recommend it to a friend
- 95% of callers followed at least some of the advice they were given, with 89% saying that they followed all of it. (Press release 2001/0113, p.1)

6 **Patient records:** two pilots launched allowing patients in two GP practices online access to their own records.

**Cancer:** Government accepts recommendations in report from National Radiological Protection Board on links between electromagnetic fields and cancer.

This found that the risk of leukaemia is doubled in those aged under 15 if exposed to electromagnetic radiation for prolonged periods.

**12 Medicines:** first steps towards a national Medicines Management Service announced. Health authorities, primary care groups and trusts invited to make bids to run first wave of sites. The aim is for:

- improvements in health through improved medicines management, using accepted markers
- a reduction in the wastage of medicines
- a reduction in unmet, evidence-based pharmaceutical need in at least one priority therapeutic area
- an improvement in medicines taking through the development of patient partnerships
- a reduction in the inappropriate clerical and professional time taken up with existing medicines management processes (e.g. in repeat prescribing)
- improved patient satisfaction with the medicines management services provided. (Press release 2001/0107, p.2; www.doh.gov.uk/pharmacyfuture /mmsection1.htm)

**Drug misuse:** £25 million announced to be used to reduce drug deaths and improve services for drug users.

**13 Staff recruitment:** £135 million announced for recruiting more nurses and GPs. The measures include:

- a £5000 'golden hello' for every new GP who joins the NHS
- a payment of up to £5000 for every GP on the retainer scheme who returns to NHS work, either part time or full time

- a £10,000 'golden handcuffs' for GPs who wait until their 65th birthday to retire from the NHS
- an additional £5000 for newly qualified GPs who go to work in deprived areas and those where there are few doctors per head of population (on top of the £5000 for every new GP)
- a 10.4% boost in bursaries for student nurses, midwives and therapists – equivalent to £500 for England's 48,000 nursing diploma students and £200 for its 22,000 nursing degree students
- £1000 for all nurses, midwives and therapists who undertake return to practice courses
- £15 million to provide 50 more NHS workplace nurseries (on top of the extra 100 already planned). (Press release 2001/0128, p.1)

**14 Smoking cessation services:** nicotine replacement therapies to be made available on prescription, and certain nicotine patches, lozenges and gums allowed on general sale.

**16 Prescription charges:** charge raised from £6.00 to £6.10, the lowest rate of increase for 20 years.

**NHS Direct:** two pilot digital TV projects launched that will provide interactive services between homes and NHS Direct advice and information.

**17 General practice:** £100 million a year allocated to the improvement of primary care, to be allocated as follows:

- a lump sum of approximately £5000 will be paid up-front to help practices provide improved services

– such as extra clinics, extended opening hours, training GP specialists and better heart and cancer services. Primary care groups (PCGs) and primary care trusts (PCTs) will draw up with practices their own incentive schemes that will deliver local improvements to reflect NHS priorities

- the second tranche of cash will be paid out at the end of the financial year, provided that the practice hits its local incentive targets. Practices hitting the targets will have complete freedom to spend the subsequent bonus. GPs can take it as a cash sum for themselves, reward practice staff or put the money back into patient services. (Press release 2001/0138, p.1)

**19 Winter planning:** report published on NHS performance during winter 2000/01. It concluded that:

- the planning for winter had been effective, with very good joint working between health and social care
- the promotion of health and self-care had been good, with successful flu immunisation and self-care programmes, and the extension of NHS Direct across the country
- despite low flu levels, the demand for hospital services had been *higher* than last year, with increased numbers of emergency admissions and ambulance call-outs
- additionally, primary care and social care came under particular pressures, including losses of residential and nursing home places in some parts of the country, heavy flooding and bad weather
- these increased pressures had been handled well: there had been fewer

patients waiting for long periods on trolleys, fewer operations cancelled at the last minute, fewer delayed discharges, additional services provided to people in their own homes, additional acute and critical care beds, and additional staff

- the pressures had been managed successfully due to the hard work and determination of people throughout the system, supported by additional resources and new ways of planning and working.

**20 Learning disabilities:** new strategy launched based on civil rights, independence, choice and inclusion. Specific initiatives include:

- a new Learning Disability Development Fund of up to £100 million over the next two years
- an end to long-stay hospitals by helping people move to more appropriate accommodation in the community
- specialist local services for people with severe challenging behaviour and developing integrated facilities for children with severe disabilities and complex needs
- a five-year programme to modernise local council day services
- a new £6 million Implementation Support Fund over the next three years to fund new advocacy developments and a national learning disability information centre and helpline in partnership with Mencap
- a £2 million learning disability research initiative
- the first ever national objectives for services for people with learning disabilities, supported by new targets and performance indicators
- more choice and control for people

with learning disabilities by extended eligibility to direct payments, establishing a National Citizen Advocacy Network and increasing funding for self-advocacy organisations, in partnership with the voluntary sector

- a new national forum for people with learning disabilities
- the creation of a Learning Disability Task Force
- a Learning Disability Awards Framework to provide a new qualification route for care workers. (Press release 2001/0140, p.2)

**25 Immunisation:** immunisation against tuberculosis restarted, the programme having been suspended in 1999 due to manufacturing difficulties.

**26 Cancer:** National Cancer Research Institute to be launched on 1 April. The Institute will:

> … co-ordinate all cancer research in the UK. It will bring together all UK Health Departments, the Medical Research Council, the Cancer Research Campaign, Imperial Cancer Research Fund, the Ludwig Institute for Cancer Research, the Marie Curie Research Institute, and the pharmaceutical industry. (Press release 2001/0149, p.1)

In addition, £6 million announced for the development of two centres of excellence for prostate cancer research.

**27 Old people:** *National Service Framework for Older People* published. It embodies eight standards covering:

- rooting out age discrimination
- person-centred care

- intermediate care
- general hospital care
- stroke
- falls
- mental health in older people
- the promotion of health and active life in older age. (HSC 2001/017, p.3)

The Standing Nursing and Midwifery Advisory Committee published *Caring for Older People: A Nursing Priority*, which focuses on care for older people in acute settings.

**28 Pharmaceuticals:** report of the Pharmaceutical Industry Competitiveness Task Force published, setting out proposed action in a range of areas:

- the role that intellectual property rights (IPR) and the TRIPs agreement play, and should continue to play, in the flow of innovative medicines. One of the most important outputs of the Task Force is the renewed industry … to work towards improving access to medicines in developing countries
- streamlining licensing procedures for essential research involving animals has been agreed, cutting red tape and improving animal welfare. This complements amendments to the Criminal Justice and Police Bill and Malicious Communications Act to tackle harassment and intimidation by animal rights campaigners
- a more forward-looking strategic dialogue about developments in health care and the market for medicines in the UK
- involving the industry closely in the development of NHS services.
- agreement that new policy

measures should not be viewed in isolation, but as part of the overall environment

- industry and government agreed positions on a range of medicines' policy issues under discussion in the European Union
- indicators of performance and competitiveness that will allow government and industry to measure and monitor the progress of the UK as a competitive location for pharmaceutical investment. (Press release 2001/0155, p.2)

**Health checks:** pilot schemes for health checks on retirement launched.

29 **E-prescribing:** three pilots approved to test risks, benefits and costs of transmitting prescriptions electronically.

30 **Medical training:** two medical schools announced at Exeter and Plymouth, and the University of East Anglia, and 1003 extra medical places. The intention is to open up opportunities to those from middle- and lower-income families.

## APRIL

1 **Medicines:** £1.3 million announced:

> ... to support the work of a national joint task force which will bring together representatives of patients, the NHS, social care, health professions and the pharmaceutical industry. The funds will support a project team, based at the Royal Pharmaceutical Society of Great Britain, which will work under the direction of the task force. (Press release 2001/0166, p.1)

4 **Hospitals:** *Implementing the NHS Plan – Modern Matrons* (HSC 2001/010) requires the role of all ward sisters and charge nurses to be strengthened so that there is a:

> ... highly visible, accessible and authoritative figure upon whom patients can rely to ensure that the fundamentals of care are right.

There are three main strands to the matron role:

- securing and assuring the highest standards of clinical care by providing leadership to the professional and direct care staff within the group of wards for which they are accountable
- ensuring that administrative and support services are designed and delivered to achieve the highest standards of care within the group of wards for which they are accountable
- providing a visible, accessible and authoritative presence in ward settings to whom patients and their families can turn for assistance, advice and support. (p.6)

5 **Exercise:** national standards for GP exercise referral schemes published. The programmes will include patients with:

- coronary heart disease/hypertension, obesity and diabetes
- mental health problems, including depression
- musculo-skeletal problems, such as chronic low-back pain
- rehabilitation following falls and accidents, particularly among the elderly. (Press release 2001/0177, p.1)

6 **Mental health:** £30 million announced for improving wards for psychiatric patients.

9 **Cancer:** large-scale trial announced, to be funded by the Department of Health, comparing monitoring, radical prostatectomy and radical radiotherapy.

10 **Dentistry:** the Continuing Professional Development Scheme announced, designed to compensate dentists for loss of earnings while undergoing continuing professional education.

12 **Walk-in centres:** three more walk-in centres announced, bringing the total to 43 since the first were established in July 1999.

17 **Quality of care:** National Patient Safety Agency announced in *Building a Safer NHS for Patients*. The Agency will:

- collect and analyse information on adverse events from local NHS organisations, NHS staff and patients and carers
- assimilate other safety-related information from a variety of existing reporting systems and other sources in this country and abroad
- learn lessons and ensure that they are fed back into practice, service organisation and delivery
- produce solutions to prevent harm where risks are identified, and set out national goals and establish ways of tracking progress towards these goals. (Press release 2001/0190, p.2)

19 **Genetics:** in the first speech on genetics by a health secretary, a five-point plan for improvement of genetic services announced, comprising:

- by 2006, the number of specialist consultants in genetics will double from 77 to 140
- the number of NHS scientific and technical staff working in genetics will rise by 300 over the next five years
- the number of specialist genetic counsellors working in the NHS will increase by at least 150
- two new national laboratories for genetics will be set up to specialise in rare genetic disorders and diseases, and identify new tests and treatments that can bring benefits to patients
- NHS genetics services will be reorganised into a single national network to make sure all NHS patients get the same standard of specialist genetic services, regardless of where they happen to live. (Press release 2001/0194, p.1)

23 **Child poverty:** £40 million over three years announced to help reduce child poverty and improve health in rural areas. The funding is to be used to extend services and support already available via Sure Start.

25 **NHS structure:** Secretary of State sets out plans to 'hand power to frontline staff'. The proposals require that:

- by 2004, two-thirds of the 99 health authorities will have merged – devolving many of their responsibilities to primary care trusts (PCTs). The 30 'strategic health authorities' that remain will cover a larger section of the population

- health authorities will have responsibility devolved to them from the eight NHS regional offices for performance managing the local health care system
- the new strategic health authorities will provide the bridge between the Department of Health and local NHS services, brokering solutions to local problems, holding local health services to account and encouraging greater autonomy for NHS trusts and primary care trusts. The best performing NHS organisations will be invited to bid to run the new strategic health authorities. (Press release 2001/ 0200, p.1)

30 **Screening:** new screening programmes for cystic fibrosis and hearing impairment announced.

**MAY**

2 **Medicines:** new set of best practice guidelines issued to protect patients when drugs are withdrawn from the market.

**Maternity care:** £100 million announced for maternity services to be spent on:

- new single-room provision providing more privacy for families
- more comfortable rooms with home comforts like televisions and telephones
- rooms provided for fathers to stay, especially where babies need special care.

It was also announced that a national service framework for children and maternity services will include new standards to ensure that:

- women will have access to a midwife dedicated to them when in established labour 100% of the time
- all women will have access to care delivered by midwives they know and trust
- an end to the lottery in child birth choices – so that women in all parts of the country, not just some, have greater choice, including the choice of a safe home birth. (Press release 2001/0212)

It was also announced that a new national service framework is to be established for children and maternity services.

3 **Air pollution:** Committee on the Medical Effects of Air Pollutants publishes estimates of the health effects of long-term exposure to particulate air pollution.

**Dentistry:** review of dental workforce announced, following report from the Health Select Committee.

4 **Dentistry:** £35 million announced for dental services to be used for:

- refurbishing and redecorating surgeries and waiting areas for the benefit of patients
- buying new dental equipment to encourage up-to-date treatments
- improving disabled access and installing play areas for children
- installing new IT systems to speed up appointments and recall systems. (Press release 2001/0219, p.1)

6 **Hospitals:** £105 million allocated for new hospital equipment.

8 **Hospitals:** new menu for NHS hospitals announced, offering more

choice, more fresh food, and more options for vegetarian and other specialist diets.

**Dentistry:** range of treatments available to non-registered patients extended following Select Committee report.

# The battle for public opinion

Jo-Ann Mulligan

For a government sensitive to the ebbs and flows in public opinion, the state of the NHS is a hazardous subject. A series of scandals has created the impression of a health service often near the brink of crisis and occasionally a name (Mavis Skeet, Harold Shipman, Rodney Ledwood …) conjures up an image of all that is apparently wrong with the service. In fact, the reality is often more mundane, and most people are broadly happy with the service they get from the NHS. However, Londoners may feel they have more reason than most to voice concern, and there is no doubt that London's health service faces special challenges: for instance, the continuing struggle with ageing hospital buildings, shortages of key staff, and patchy primary care services. So what do Londoners make of health care in the capital? How do they view Labour's first four years? And what can we say about their expectations for the future of the NHS?

The King's Fund and the *Evening Standard* jointly commissioned a survey in February 2001 to explore Londoners' attitudes towards health and health care in the capital (see Box 1). The survey interviewed people across Greater London about their views on hospital and GP services, their use of the private sector, and attitudes towards suggested alternatives to the NHS. Inevitably, perceptions of performance are bound up with the politics of the NHS, particularly in an election year. Therefore, where relevant, we also examine the party allegiance of respondents.

## BOX 1: KING'S FUND/EVENING STANDARD SURVEY

The King's Fund/*Evening Standard* survey was conducted by ICM Research with a team of professional telephone interviewers using a structured interview schedule. ICM interviewed a random sample of 1000 adults, aged 18 and over, between 23 and 25 February 2001. Quotas were applied to standard demographics to ensure that the sample was representative of London as a whole, and the results were weighted to the profile of all adults.

## QUALITY OF HEALTH SERVICES

A key objective of any health system is to deliver good quality services to the population. At first sight, the signs are encouraging: a majority of Londoners (57 per cent) believe that when they reach hospital they can be confident of obtaining high-quality treatment (see Table 1 below). Interestingly, public confidence in the quality of services provided by GPs appears consistently higher than that provided by hospitals – a substantial majority (72 per cent) thought they would get high-quality GP services (see Table 2 below).

Londoners with recent NHS experience (those who told ICM they had been outpatients or inpatients within the last two years) were slightly *less* likely to feel confident of getting high-quality hospital treatment than those without experience (55 per cent vs 60 per cent). This is intriguing, as evidence from other surveys suggest that it is those *without* recent NHS experience who tend to express negative views. Our finding could be an effect peculiar to London: evidence from other surveys (though not fully explaining this result) suggests that Londoners tend to be more critical of health services than people elsewhere.[1] Of course, an alternative explanation is that negative perceptions of the NHS are grounded in actual experience.

Asking people the more political question of whether services had *improved* over the past four years elicits more worrying results. Only 15 per cent of respondents thought hospital services had improved and just over a third believed things had got worse. Attitudes towards GPs were again more favourable, with 25 per cent saying things had improved, against 16 per cent who thought things had got worse. Clearly, attitudes towards the health service are influenced by many

## Table 1: If I had to go to hospital, I would feel confident of getting high-quality treatment on the NHS

|  | Recent hospital experience | | |
|  | All % | Yes % | No % |
|---|---|---|---|
| Agree | 57 | 55 | 60 |
| Disagree | 39 | 42 | 37 |
| Base | *1000* | *498* | *502* |

## Table 2: If I had to see my GP, I would feel confident of getting high-quality treatment

|  | Recent GP experience | | |
|  | All % | Yes % | No % |
|---|---|---|---|
| Agree | 72 | 73 | 69 |
| Disagree | 26 | 26 | 26 |
| Base | *1000* | *847* | *153* |

factors other than direct experience of the health service. In particular, public expectations and the prevailing political climate are often strongly associated with opinion poll findings. When the above results are broken down by political allegiance (as measured by voting intentions), it is Labour supporters who

## Figure 1: Political allegiance and attitudes towards the NHS

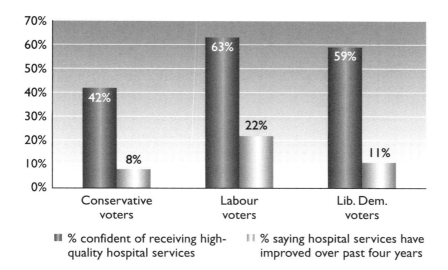

■ % confident of receiving high-quality hospital services

■ % saying hospital services have improved over past four years

## Figure 2: Sources of Information about the NHS

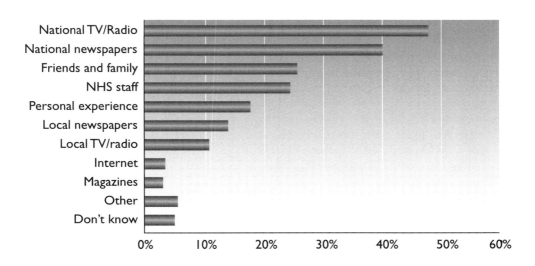

## Table 3: How long does it normally take to obtain a non-urgent appointment to see your GP, or another doctor at the same surgery?

|  | 2001 Social class | | | 1999 Social class | | |
|---|---|---|---|---|---|---|
|  | All | ABC1 | C2DE | All | ABC1 | C2DE |
|  | % | % | % | % | % | % |
| Same day | 20 | 18 | 23 | 21 | 18 | 24 |
| Next day | 12 | 12 | 13 | 18 | 17 | 19 |
| Within three days | 23 | 24 | 20 | 27 | 27 | 28 |
| Longer than three days | 36 | 37 | 34 | 28 | 33 | 23 |
| Base | 1000 | 599 | 401 | 1002 | 522 | 480 |

are more likely be confident of obtaining high-quality hospital services and who believe that the NHS has improved over the last four years. It seems asking people how they feel about the NHS turns out to be as much a question about the performance of the government of the day as it is about the performance of the health service.

Given the variety of factors that potentially influence opinions, it is useful to know the sources people rely on for information about the NHS. We asked respondents to name their top two sources. As Figure 2 shows, almost half (48 per cent) said that television and radio was one of their top two sources of information about the NHS. Newspapers were also cited by 40 per cent, and friends and family by 26 per cent. Nearly one in four cited NHS staff, usually their GP. Personal experience was mentioned by 18 per cent of respondents. Only 3 per cent per cent mentioned the Internet as a main source of information.

### ACCESS TO HEALTH SERVICES

Previous polls have shown that the public's main concern about the NHS is

waiting – waiting to see a GP, waiting to see a consultant, and waiting for treatment. In contrast to the questions that seek opinions about the health service, we also asked a question about Londoners' *experience* of the health service. One in five Londoners said they would be able to get a non-urgent appointment with their GP on the same day (see Table 3 above). However, the majority of people (59 per cent) would have to wait more than two days, and more than a third (36 per cent) said they would have to wait more than three days to see a GP. The same question was asked by the King's Fund in 1999, and a comparison of results suggests that access to GPs has not improved over the last two years.[2] Most notably, the proportion waiting more than three days to see any doctor has increased from 28 per cent to 36 per cent.

Some people reported finding it easier to get appointments than others. Nearly a quarter (23 per cent) of those in social classes C2DE said they could get an appointment on the same day, compared with 18 per cent of those in social classes ABC1. This apparently counter-intuitive

# Table 4: Private medical insurance and household income

| | All | Household income | | |
| | | Less than £20,000 | £20–40,000 | £40,000 and over |
| | % | % | % | % |
|---|---|---|---|---|
| Has private medical insurance | 28 | 14 | 33 | 51 |
| ... employer pays majority of the cost | 63 | 41 | 61 | 75 |
| Has paid for a medical consultation | 23 | 19 | 22 | 29 |
| Has paid for hospital treatment | 10 | 7 | 10 | 14 |
| *Base* | *1000* | *345* | *252* | *213* |

result is also seen in other surveys by the Department of Health and the King's Fund.[3,4] One explanation could be related to the perceived urgency of visits: evidence from elsewhere suggests that patients from higher socio-economic groups are less likely to consider the reason for their visit to be urgent than those in lower social groups.[5]

## PRIVATE HEALTH CARE

People who are disenchanted with the NHS can, if they can afford it, take out private medical insurance (PMI). Over a quarter of Londoners now have some form of private health insurance plan (28 per cent). This appears to be greater than that for Britain as a whole: the latest *British Social Attitudes* survey (using more or less the same definition) found that 19 per cent of the population had some sort of private health insurance.[6] Of course, possession of PMI does not mean people necessarily always use it. For the many people who have private health insurance, combined use of private and public medical services is the norm.[7]

In addition to private health insurance, a significant minority of Londoners also pay for private health care out of their own pockets: 23 per cent of respondents had paid for a private medical consultation in the UK and 10 per cent had had private hospital treatment. Predictably, use of the private sector appears to be strongly related to household income, to the extent that over half of Londoners with a household income of over £40,000 have private medical insurance.

## THE FUTURE OF THE NHS

Finally, we asked Londoners about their attitudes to different 'futures' for the NHS. Opinion polls about future changes to the NHS rarely, if ever, distinguish between what people would like to see change and how likely such change is to come about. Separating out opinions about what *ought* to change from what *will* change can be revealing. To explore this, the poll posed five statements about possible changes in the way the NHS is funded and organised, and asked members of the public whether they supported or opposed these changes. We also asked respondents how likely (or unlikely) they thought these various developments were to occur in the next ten years. The results revealed some big differences between what the public would like to see change and what they think will actually change during that period (Table 5).

Overall, public attitudes in London towards the NHS, and suggested alternatives, are not straightforward. On the one hand, opposition to a two-tier NHS remains high (75 per cent), regardless of age, income or political allegiance. Yet a substantial minority of Londoners (42 per cent) also believes that the Government should encourage the take-up of private health insurance. It seems that, while respondents feel that universal free care should be available, they nevertheless feel that people should also have the choice to buy private medical care.

Labour remains hostile to expansion of private health insurance, but the NHS Plan signalled a warmer relationship with the private sector in terms of provision.[8] Our results, however, indicate that the Government may need to proceed with caution on this issue in the capital: only 37 per cent supported the NHS relying less on its own hospitals, and this fell to 34 per cent among Labour supporters. Despite these concerns, many Londoners believe greater private sector involvement is inevitable. Seven in ten said the Government is likely to encourage a greater take-up of PMI, and six in ten felt it likely that the NHS would rely less on its own hospitals over the next ten years and purchase more care from the private sector.

The finding that four in ten respondents are opposed to the NHS remaining the same and 50 per cent support an earmarked health tax is perhaps not

## Table 5: Options for the NHS

|  | Strongly support or tend to support | Strongly oppose or tend to oppose | Very or fairly likely to happen | Very or fairly unlikely to happen |
|---|---|---|---|---|
| Government. to encourage take-up of private medical insurance | 42 | 54 | 73 | 22 |
| NHS to rely less on its own hospitals and to pay private sector to do more work | 37 | 59 | 62 | 31 |
| Cut taxes, and leave NHS for emergencies and the poor only | 21 | 75 | 38 | 57 |
| Hypothecated NHS tax | 50 | 39 | 40 | 47 |
| Funding and organisation of NHS to stay more or less as it is now | 54 | 41 | 64 | 30 |

Base = 1000

surprising. In fact, the latter attracted the least opposition of the five options offered. They could both reflect a more general frustration with the pace of change in the NHS and reveal at least a modest desire to experiment with different ways of organising and even of funding services.

Interestingly, possession of PMI appears to be associated with particular views about the future of the health service. For instance, those with PMI are less likely to be confident of receiving high-quality NHS care and (unsurprisingly) are more likely to support government-backed expansion of PMI. Of course, it is impossible to tell from these data the direction of causation. Does possession of PMI mean people are more likely to be critical of the NHS or vice versa? Individuals with PMI may see themselves as paying twice for health and so be more likely to resist increases in taxation to spend on health. This might imply that a growing private sector will eventually undermine support for the NHS. Yet, according to our poll, possession of PMI does not preclude support for the principle of a universal NHS: 71 per cent of those with PMI are still opposed to the idea of the NHS being kept only for emergencies and the poor. Trend data from the *British Social Attitudes* survey suggests that possession of private health insurance may have more to do with the state of the economy rather than any significant shift in attitudes towards the NHS.[9] This is plausible given that the majority of those with insurance have it paid for by their employer. In addition, many people with PMI are still reliant on the NHS for certain types of care, most notably primary care and emergency care. Nevertheless, although the private sector for the UK as a whole has remained more or less static over the last decade, the impact of increases in private medical insurance coverage on public support for the NHS in the future remains uncertain.

## CONCLUSIONS

Opinion polls are fraught with methodological difficulties and it is important not to over-interpret findings. The intention here is to provide a snapshot of the overall *mood* of Londoners towards the health service in an election year, rather than provide a definitive account of experiences of the NHS.

Londoners remain firmly in support of a tax-funded NHS, and radical moves in the direction of restricting the scope of the NHS risks offending public opinion, regardless of political persuasion. On the other hand, the public appears more prepared to accept new ways of financing the NHS from the public purse. For instance, hypothecated taxes are supported by over half of those living in the capital; however, the extent to which earmarked taxes represent a viable way of funding the NHS is still unclear.

In their audit of the Government's performance, Polly Toynbee and David Walker concluded that Labour 'is left with a weak record on health only able to promise that the best is yet to come over the second term'.[10] Eventually, Labour will have to make good on that promise and some argue that leaving the bulk of spending to the second term is a risky strategy. Nevertheless, while Londoners may have detected little improvement in services, they still believe that it is Labour, not the Conservatives, who currently has the best policies on health.[11] The challenge for Labour's second term must be to deliver on the promises made in its first term, whilst moderating the public's burgeoning expectations. That trick may yet prove impossible.

## REFERENCES

1 Judge J, Solomon M. Public opinion and the National Health Service: patterns and perspectives in consumer satisfaction. *Journal of Social Policy* 1993; 22 (3): 299–327.

2 Malbon G, Jenkins C, Gillam S. *What do Londoners think of their general practice?* London: King's Fund, 1999.

3 *Ibid.*

4 Department of Health. *National survey of NHS patients. General practice 1998.* London: NHS Executive, 1999.

5 *Ibid.*

6 Jowell R, Curtice J, Park A *et al.*, editors. *British social attitudes. The 17th report.* London: Sage, 2000.

7 Emmerson C, Frayne, C, Goodman A. Should private medical insurance be subsidised? In: Appleby J, Harrison A, editors. *Health Care UK Spring 2001.* London: King's Fund, 2001.

8 Secretary of State for Health. *The new NHS: modern, dependable.* Cm 3807. London: Stationery Office, 1997.

9 Mulligan J. Attitudes towards the NHS and its alternatives. In: Harrison A, editor. *Health Care UK 1997/98.* London: King's Fund, 1998.

10 Toynbee P, Walker D. *Did things get better? An audit of Labour's successes and failures.* London: Penguin, 2001.

11 Kellner P. Capital's hopes tied up with Labour. *Evening Standard* 2001; 1 March: 8.

# Mental health services in London

Angela Greatley

Mental health professionals and users have for many years argued for greater priority to be given to mental health services in Britain. Recently, new initiatives such as the national service framework (NSF) for mental health, elements of the NHS Plan and the Policy Implementation Guide, have set out the kind of mental health service that we should expect and emphasise the high priority that government gives to achieving change. However, the history of delivering change in mental health care at local level is not a happy one, with great variability in the range and quality of services across the country. It has also proved very difficult to obtain the kind of information that allows progress (or the lack of it) to be monitored systematically. A key requirement now that there is a clear national strategy and goals is the need to be able to track the proposed changes in mental health services.

## BACKGROUND

The NSF for mental health was one of the earliest frameworks.[1] Published at the end of 1999, there was significant support among professionals, users and carers for the values and principles that underpin it, as well as for the programme it set out for developments in planning and service delivery.

Setting quality standards in five areas of mental health, it provides models both for promoting health and treating illness. It deals with the need for the development of high-quality services of known effectiveness and for much greater involvement of individuals in planning their own care and of user groups in planning services. It emphasises the importance of tackling social exclusion and of improving quality of life for people with mental health problems, creating non-discriminatory services that promote independence and are supported by well-co-ordinated health and social care partnerships. It also points out the problems created by a legacy of poor-quality information in both mental health care and social services, and the need for improvement in this area in order to record and measure change effectively.

In London, the NHS Executive and the Social Services Inspectorate produced a strategy for London's mental health,[2] following wide consultations and discussions within London's mental health community. The strategy emphasises that mental health is about quality of life. It also notes that care and treatment are only one element in the lives of service users, and highlights the importance of friendships, financial security, adequate housing, work and leisure for people with mental health

## BOX 1: NEW ELEMENTS OF THE COMMUNITY MENTAL HEALTH SERVICES

- **Assertive outreach** offering comprehensive community-based care, practical support and high-quality treatment for the most seriously ill people who will not engage with services and who often lead relatively chaotic lives; an assertive outreach team is multidisciplinary and offers intensive and frequent contact on the users' own terms.
- **Crisis resolution** offering home treatments for those with acute mental health problems, many of whom would otherwise find themselves in hospital; a crisis resolution team is multidisciplinary and works with users and their carers until the crisis has been resolved and less intense community services are sufficient.
- **Early intervention teams** working specifically with young people who show signs of the onset of what may become a serious mental illness; the multidisciplinary team works to offer expert treatment and care to promote recovery and to work for inclusion.

problems. The strategy also emphasises the importance of relevant and appropriate information if users and professionals are to be able to assess progress.

In addition to the NSF, the NHS Plan[3] has made mental health one of its three clinical priorities, and sets out both investment and objectives to be achieved. Some of the Plan's milestones are quite specific and set within relatively short timescales – for example, the completion of the programme to create a network of assertive outreach, crisis resolution and early intervention teams (see Box 1 above). Other objectives need significantly more flesh on the bones – for example, more detail is required about proposals for a new kind of primary care mental health worker. Overall, all the targets set by the NHS Plan are ambitious and delivery will rely on new ways of working – for instance, by working in new forms of partnership between health, social care and other agencies. Implementation will also require significant amounts of new money, in addition to better use of all resources already within mental health.

Earlier this year, the Department of Health issued a Policy Implementation Guide[4] bringing together guidance arising from the NSF and the Plan, together with detailed arrangements for monitoring change. When the guide was launched earlier this year, there was some surprise at the degree of specificity about the required components in a community mental health service and worries that the bigger picture might get lost. Dr Matt Muijen of the Sainsbury Centre summed this up by emphasising that, while there are many exciting service elements planned, there is also a need for someone 'to integrate the systems elements ... and guide the service user'.[5]

## IMPLEMENTING CHANGE IN MENTAL HEALTH

The initiatives and plans described above were, at least in part, a reaction to patchy and poor quality in mental health care. What has sometimes been called 'locally driven and locally owned development' has actually been a recipe for variation, with gaps in service and confusion for users and their carers. For London, this has been a particularly depressing scene. When the King's Fund's London

Commission considered the capital's mental health services in the mid-1990s, the picture was indeed gloomy. The report to the Commission, *London's Mental Health*, was published in 1997[6] and it described extreme variation, great pressure on resources, gaps in service and often poor quality across the capital's mental health services.

The report pointed to a crisis in mental health care in inner London and to many problems in outer London and in other urban mental health services. The picture painted five years ago was one of pockets of good practice barely discernible within a generally gloomy environment. As the report said: 'No single service appears to have a full range of desirable features.' There was very little 'evidence or guidance available to local planners'.

Government has made it clear across the whole of the NHS that with extra investment comes the need for assurance that appropriate services will be developed and sustained throughout the country. But the right kind of information is also needed to assess change and to measure how far services achieve developments that really matter to users and that affect their quality of life.

It has often been hard to implement mental health policy development, but it has been equally hard to measure progress, with poor information and a regrettable tendency for the services to 'tick the boxes' rather than tackle the major problems. The introduction of the Care Programme Approach was the 1990s salutary lesson on that score. Government introduced a requirement for individual care planning for service users in 1991 and progress was regularly monitored. However, this became a paper exercise in many places, and by the time

the NSF was published, though examples of long-standing good practice were offered, it was still necessary to specify what should be in a good care plan.

## INFORMATION FOR ASSESSMENT AND EVALUATION OF NEW INITIATIVES

Despite the progress that has been made on some fronts (for example, in the development of policy and in plans for implementation) many questions remain. Key among these is the question of whether we have the right kind of information to assess progress in achieving change.

The King's Fund, the Sainsbury Centre for Mental Health and the Department of Health have sponsored the 'Working Together in London' programme. Beginning in 1998, the work was devised partly in response to the findings of *London's Mental Health*. 'Working Together' explores how far the introduction of assertive outreach services can create 'more inclusive' mental health care for the people with the most severe and complex problems. Evaluation of the programme will be complete at the end of this year.

As part of the programme, the King's Fund and the Sainsbury Centre have undertaken preliminary work to show how far progress is being made towards achieving a better quality of life for service users. But this is proving difficult to measure because there are few existing and agreed methods. User-led monitoring has been incorporated within the evaluation plan. The team will interview individuals who are using the services in an attempt to measure outcomes for those individuals. This will form part of the evaluation of the programme but could also contribute to national thinking about the best way of monitoring change – using the vital information supplied by users themselves.

## CONCLUSIONS

The agreement represented in the national service framework was hard won. It has provided the map of where mental health services can get to if they tackle identified service deficits and play their part in meeting a broader range of needs – for housing, for education, for employment and for leisure. There is a growing body of research evidence including, most importantly, evidence from users about what works well for them. We know that achieving the changes needed will involve moving on both specific, shorter-term goals, and on the broader framework if services are to avoid fragmentation.

Mental health service planners and providers need more appropriate information about specific service changes if they are to measure progress. For example, hospital admission and re-admission rates are collected, but how are they to be interpreted? If admission rates rise following the introduction of an assertive outreach team, should service planners assume this is a problem? In fact, when a team is working effectively, it generally means that people in the greatest need have actually been identified and offered treatment. Subsequent admissions for those individuals are likely to be shorter in length and less frequent, with planned episodes only when necessary.

A great deal of monitoring information is gathered: NSF implementation plans, performance assessment frameworks and best value indicators for social services and key statistical returns for health, among others. However, these often assess progress on delivering the infrastructure and still fall short of measuring progress in creating an effective system. Strategic change remains difficult to measure.

At an individual level, a great deal of information is gathered about episodes of care or contacts with services. But this falls short of measuring the progress of individuals through the system and assessing the extent to which they have received appropriate care, treatment and support. There is a great deal further to go to find ways of measuring whether individuals' experiences of health care are appropriate and yet further to see whether they are helped to find a job, and then supported to stay in work, or if mental health services find them adequate housing and help them to pay the rent and keep up the tenancy – all the things, in fact, that contribute to the quality of individuals' lives.

Mental health services have now been given greater priority by government, plus new resources. Clearer central guidance has been offered (even though its specificity has not been welcomed universally by managers and professionals in local services). Mental health services need to address the agenda that has been set and cannot afford to get it wrong by failing to implement policy effectively, or leaving the gaps in provision, or failing to improve poor-quality services. However, the Centre must find innovative ways of assessing progress, moving away from measuring episodes and contacts to measures that can actually help to demonstrate whether users are getting a better deal from services and have a higher quality of life.

## REFERENCES

1 Department of Health. *A national service framework for mental health*. London: Department of Health, 1999.

2 NHS Executive. *A strategy for action*. London: NHS Executive and Social Services Inspectorate, 2000.

3 Department of Health. *The NHS Plan: a plan for investment; a plan for reform*. Cm 4818-I. London: The Stationery Office, 2000.

4 Department of Health. *Mental health policy implementation guide*. London: Department of Health, 2001.

5 Muijen M. Plans not ready for take-off. *Health Service Journal* 2001; 12 April: 20.

6 Johnson S *et al*. *London's mental health: the report to the King's Fund Commission*. London: King's Fund, 1997.

# Asylum seekers' and refugees' health experience

## Naaz Coker

Published research and stories from refugees – and health professionals who provide care to refugees – highlight the significant health needs of this group, and frequently reflect the traumas they experienced in their countries of origin, the difficult journeys they may have made, and the exclusion they experience on arrival in the UK.

Some of the health problems are clearly associated with the atrocities experienced in their own countries, such as physical trauma and injuries through torture, mental health problems including post-traumatic stress disorder, nutritional deficiencies, infection, and the lack of immunisations among young children.

### LIBUSE'S STORY (A ROMA ASYLUM SEEKER)

Under Communism my husband always had work; he worked as a roofer. When democracy came, he lost his job. We had three children. Under democracy, people know they can do and say terrible things to us. Nobody will stop them and there is nobody to defend us. On buildings, you see graffiti: 'Send the gypsies to the gas chambers'; 'Gypsies go back to India'. In shops, we got sold bad meat or rotting vegetables. On the street, people would spit on us.

Some skinheads broke into our home. It was after midnight. Ten men broke the door down and got inside. Three of them got hold of my husband – two were holding him and one hitting him. The children woke up and started screaming. One of the men hit me and I fell down. To stop my children screaming, one held a gun to my daughter's head. Next, two of them grabbed me. They held me down and another three raped me. After that they went. I was covered in a lot of blood and had terrible stomach pains. We didn't want to go the police because we were worried it would happen again. After about a week, I was in such terrible pain that we went to hospital. I didn't tell them what had happened. I had to have a hysterectomy. After that I had a mental breakdown. I was taking medication. Even now if I see a man in leather trousers, I get a panic attack.

We decided we had no choice but to leave. We came in summer 1997 and asked for asylum in Dover. We spent three days in a detention centre. Our asylum was refused at first, but after an appeal we got a year's leave to stay here. We have a flat now, but work very hard to pay the rent. We both have health problems and I worry a lot about my mother and sister back home in Slovakia.

In exile, they suffer from separation and loss of family and friends, community and cultural reference points. Homesickness coupled with anxiety and guilt about those they have left behind create further stresses. These are further compounded by lengthy asylum procedures, fear of deportation, poverty and homelessness, especially if they do not wish to be dispersed.

Many refugees will not have had access to medical help in their own countries due to war, persecution or natural disaster. Refugee women are in an even more vulnerable situation. They may have been subjected to rape, torture and sexual abuse, resulting in both physical and mental complications. The thought of being examined by a male doctor will deter many from seeking medical help. This can be compounded by communication problems and lack of awareness of the system. Many have complained of racial discrimination and intolerance. Cultural beliefs as well as domestic responsibilities result in them being isolated and frustrated. Many more report depression and ill health. Uptake of screening and prevention measures is low.

Refugee children will have complex needs. Many of them have suffered the same traumas and distress as their parents, who, due to their own frailty, are unable to provide the much needed parental support, leaving the children in a fragile and vulnerable state. Consequently, they are damaged both psychologically and physically.

## WHO ARE REFUGEES?

The twentieth century has seen mass population movements: wars and armed conflicts have resulted in enforced migration of civilians from the increasing number of the world's trouble spots. Almost every part of the world has been affected, from West Africa to Indonesia, Bosnia to Afghanistan. In 1971, 10 million people fled from East Pakistan (Bangladesh) into India. The Seventies also saw the expulsion of South Asians from East Africa, largely Kenya and Uganda, as well as ideological conflicts in Indochina, the Horn of Africa, Afghanistan, Central America, Mozambique and Angola. Over the last decade, we saw conflict and war in former Yugoslavia, Bosnia and Kosovo, the Rwandan genocides, the persecution of Kurds in Iraq and Turkey, and continuing conflicts in Sri Lanka, the Horn of Africa and East Timor. There has been a war in Afghanistan since 1979 and many refugees have fled their homes; for example, there are nearly 2 million Afghan refugees in Iran and 1.2 million in Pakistan. A relatively small number have sought refuge in Europe.

Holocaust survivor Rabbi Hugo Gryn said just before he died in 1996 that future historians would call the twentieth century not only the century of the great wars, but also the century of the refugee. It was a century in which whole populations were displaced through either wars, famine, or economic or political factors. It was the century of disappearances, of people helplessly seeing others who were close to them disappear over the horizon. It was the century of genocide.

At the end of the Second World War, the needs of 40 million displaced Europeans resulted in the establishment of the Office of the United Nations High Commissioner for Refugees (UNHCR), and in 1951 the UN Refugee Convention was adopted. This set out the precise definition of a refugee. The UK, along with 135 other countries, is a signatory to the Refugee Convention and its protocol, which commits all the signatories to certain obligations, including allowing any person fleeing persecution the legal right to seek asylum. This year is the fiftieth anniversary of the Convention, but the EU governments are questioning whether the spirit and wording of the Convention is still valid and wish to review its definition. The huge worry is that the proposed review is in response to self-interests of Western countries, and not necessarily on the needs of the world's refugees.

The term refugee, as defined in the 1951 UN Convention is a person who

> ... owing to well-founded fear of being persecuted for reasons of race, religion, nationality, membership of a particular social group or political opinion, is outside the country of his/her nationality and is unable to, or owing to such fear, is unwilling to avail himself of the protection of that country; or who, not having a nationality and being outside the country of his former habitual residence, as a result of such events, is unable to or, owing to such fear, is unwilling to return to it.

## REFUGEES AND DISPLACED PEOPLE

Today there are nearly 18 million refugees in the world. Of these, about 3 million have travelled to Europe including the UK. Most, however, are in poorer countries in the developing world, particularly India and Africa. Many are living in camps in developing countries, where illness and death rates are extremely high. India has given sanctuary to a large number of refugees from Tibet, Burma and Sri Lanka. War in Sierra Leone and Liberia has caused nearly 2 million people to flee from their homes into neighbouring countries. War in Angola forced over 200,000 Angolan people to move to other African countries.

Another 25 million people have fled from their homes and have gone into hiding in their home country. These groups of people are called *internally displaced* people. Their needs are the same as refugees.

It is estimated that one person in every 150 people alive today is a refugee or a displaced person. Furthermore, there is a growing body of migrants who are leaving their homes and countries to seek educational opportunities and economic prosperity.

Last year, Britain officially received 76,000 asylum applicants. Fifty per cent of them came from Iraq, Sri Lanka, former Yugoslavia, Iran, Somalia and Afghanistan – all countries experiencing continuing turmoil, conflict and serious human rights abuses. Of the 76,000 total, 31 per cent were granted refugee status or extended leave to remain. These figures do not take into account the refusals that were overturned on appeal. In 1999, the total acceptance rate was 54 per cent.

Every year about 3500 unaccompanied refugee children arrive in Britain. Most have fled from Angola, Ethiopia, Somalia, Sierra Leone, Afghanistan, former Yugoslavia and Sri Lanka. More recently, most refugee children have come from Albania and Kosovo. Many have seen their parents killed; others have become separated from their parents during wars; others have been sent away by their parents when the situation has seemed dangerous. This has been especially the case with young boys.

Along with the official new arrivals, there are also those who arrive unofficially. However, increasingly tight immigration controls in European countries can make it very hard for some people to enter legally even if they feel they have a legitimate case to do so: for example, obtaining the right papers to leave a country officially may be impossible.

## THE ASYLUM AND IMMIGRATION ACT 1999

In the UK, the most recent piece of legislation bearing on asylum seekers and refugees is the 1999 Asylum and Immigration Act. The Act is a complex piece of legislation, but there are four key aspects that impact on asylum seekers:

- **Dispersal** – all newly arrived asylum seekers are to be dispersed outside London and the South East across the UK.
- **Introduction of vouchers** – asylum seekers are entitled to the equivalent of 70 per cent of income support, to be issued as vouchers for food and other items.
- **No-choice accommodation** – asylum seekers have to accept the accommodation offered to them or they will lose their benefits.
- **A new system of support** – the Home Office has established a new administrative unit called the National Asylum Support Service (NASS) to administer and support newly arrived asylum seekers.

The effect of the 1999 Act on key determinants of asylum seekers' and refugees' health and determinants of health has not been wholly conducive. Lack of resources is a particular problem. For example, a single adult asylum seeker receives the equivalent of £36.54 in vouchers a week, £10.00 of which is exchangeable for cash. In other words, the value of the vouchers represents 70 per cent of regular income support. Vouchers can be exchanged only in certain designated shops and no cash change is given for underspending the voucher denominations. The use of vouchers can also be socially stigmatising.

Accommodation for asylum seekers is often provided in very poor-quality housing in deprived inner city areas. Even after dispersal, there are complaints about the standard of accommodation, including damp, infestation and lack of privacy.

Compulsory dispersal has proved problematic. For example, until last year the majority of asylum seekers settled in London, where they gradually established a network of support systems. Dispersal can exacerbate feelings of isolation and social exclusion.

## MANAGING HEALTH NEEDS

Managing the health needs of refugees and asylum seekers requires a focus on four main areas: access, communication and advocacy, mental health, and training of health care professionals.

### ACCESS

Asylum seekers, refugees and those with extended leave to remain have full entitlement to NHS care.[1] However, many experience problems in registering with a GP.[2] Refugees have often described their desperate search for GPs, finding some practices reluctant to register them because of high workload. As a consequence, many end up in hospital casualty departments when ill. A key problem with access is not only a lack of knowledge about NHS services, but also ignorance on the part of NHS staff about their entitlement and rights, and prejudices of health professionals that create unnecessary barriers.

Refugees need to be offered permanent registration, together with information about how the NHS works, which will enable ongoing care and access to health promotion, and preventative services including physiotherapy, dental and pharmaceutical services. Because they have the same rights to NHS care as a UK citizen, there is no special funding available to health services. However, the Department of Health has set out a model of a Local Development Scheme (LDS) for GPs and other primary care providers that allows access to additional funds in recognition of increased workload.[3] Personal medical services (PMS) schemes have also focused on health care provision for asylum seekers and refugees.

## COMMUNICATION AND ADVOCACY

Language barriers pose the single biggest problem for recently arrived asylum seekers in need of health care. Health care professionals need to ensure that, wherever possible, interpreters or trained advocates are used during consultations, as a reliance on family members or children usually results in inaccurate interpretation or incomplete information, especially when sensitive issues need to be discussed. In situations where interpreters are not available, telephone interpreting can provide a limited but useful alternative. The particular experiences of asylum seekers (which may include torture) mean that health care professionals may need to work harder to establish trust.

## MENTAL HEALTH

The experiences of refugees pre-asylum and post-exile can contribute to mental health problems. In addition, people who have been tortured or caught up in war may have seen their family members killed or tortured, and their needs will relate to that loss and bereavement. Social exclusion, isolation and racist abuse in this country can compound their problems.

People who have been subjected to torture or seen their close family and friends tortured will require specialist support. Helen Bamber, Director of the Medical Foundation for the Care of Victims of Torture, describes torture as: ' ... the act of killing a man without his dying. The perpetrator has total power; the victim is totally helpless. Being subjected to such an experience destroys the integrity of body and mind.'[4] It is well documented that many survivors of torture are initially reluctant to disclose their experiences until they begin to feel safe and secure, and trust the professionals they encounter. Referrals to appropriate clinical expertise are critical. In addition to clinical expertise, torture victims also need the social and community support of their communities in order to recover and re-experience the feelings of belonging and independence.

There is ongoing concern on the part of many agencies who work with asylum seekers and refugees that the dispersal policy will result in torture victims ending up in parts of the country where they will be denied access to the essential clinical and community network support.

## TRAINING OF HEALTH CARE PROFESSIONALS

Health professionals often do not know how best to support the needs of refugees. Primary care services are critical, yet many GPs are confused about refugees' entitlements and offer only temporary registration, leading to fragmented patterns of care. Many feel unable to give the time needed to manage refugees' health needs and are overwhelmed by their experiences.

There are many refugee community organisations that are willing and able to work with the health system in meeting refugees' specific health care needs. Many communities have organised themselves to provide health advocacy services that inform refugees about health matters and refer them to appropriate health services. The Tamil Relief Centre in Edmonton, for example, employs a women and children's health worker, whose role is to educate and inform both women and local health professionals. Several London health authorities and trusts have set up specialist services to meet refugees' needs. Camden and Islington Community Health, for instance, has a stress trauma clinic for Bosnian refugees who have experienced atrocities in their former homes.

In 1998, the Health Education Authority,[5] in its report of the Expert Working Group on Refugee Health, made a series of recommendations to promote the health of refugees and asylum seekers. These include:

- the provision of written information, in appropriate languages, about the structure of and routes of access to the NHS
- the introduction of client-held records for newly arrived refugees
- encouraging GPs to offer permanent registration to refugees
- improving the quality of interpreting services
- the establishment of multi-disciplinary primary health care teams

to deal with health needs of newly arrived asylum seekers and refugees
- the development of a guide for clinicians and health authorities on refugee health needs
- the development of cross-cultural programmes at undergraduate and postgraduate level
- the provision of culturally sensitive services by female health workers for refugee women's obstetric and sexual health needs
- the development of a culturally appropriate mental health strategy for refugees based on a multi-agency approach.

## CONCLUSIONS

There has been growing numbers of asylum seekers in the UK, largely from countries where there is civil war, persecution or human rights abuses. The lengthy and often traumatic asylum procedures undermine the health and well-being of these vulnerable communities of people. Refugees need support to rebuild their lives and regain their identity and self-esteem. Managing their health needs is a complex process requiring a sensitive approach to identifying, assessing and responding to the particular needs of specific groups of people, many of whom will be traumatised, depressed and extremely vulnerable.

Although asylum seekers have restricted and prescribed housing and cash benefits, they are entitled to both primary and secondary NHS care. Unfortunately, entitlement is not synonymous with use, and many find it difficult if not impossible to access health services when in need.

Health professionals will need training and support in order to meet the needs of these groups of people. An important component of this support includes information on the entitlements of refugees and asylum seekers to NHS services, an understanding of why people become refugees, and the circumstances from which such people have come.

**Asylum seekers:** people who have made an application for asylum in the UK.

**Exceptional Leave to Remain (ELR):** people given ELR are allowed to stay in the UK for specified period of time, ranging from one to four years.

**Indefinite Leave to Remain (ILR):** people given ILR are granted refugee status and can apply for their dependents to join them.

People with ELR or ILR status have the same entitlements to welfare benefits, health, housing, education and employment benefits as UK citizens.

## REFERENCES

1 Levenson R, Coker N. *The health of refugees: a guide for GPs*. London: King's Fund, 1999.

2 Fassil Y. Looking after the health of refugees. *BMJ* 2000; 321: 59.

3 Audit Commission. *Another country: implementing dispersal under the Asylum and Immigration Act 1999*. Abingdon: Audit Commission, 2000.

4 St George's House Trust. *Asylum seekers in Britain – responding to the challenge. Consultation report*. Berkshire, 2000.

5 Health Education Authority Expert Working Group on Refugee Health. *Promoting the health of refugees*. London: ILPA, 1998.

# Children in the capital

Ruth Tennant and Teresa Edmans

## INTRODUCTION

Despite London's relative wealth, there are stark inequalities in the life chances of children living in different parts of the city. Babies born in Tower Hamlets are nearly twice as likely to be stillborn or of low birth weight than babies born in Richmond, are three times more likely to die before reaching the age of four, six times more likely to be killed in an accident, twice as likely to be victims of crime before reaching the age of 18, nine times more likely to live in overcrowded accommodation, and five times more likely to be in a household with non-earning adults. Multiple deprivation – poverty, poor housing, low levels of educational achievement and crime – clusters in particular parts of the city, areas that also tend to demonstrate higher-than-average levels of childhood injury and accidents, low birth-weight babies, mental health problems, and teenage conception.

Since the election of a Labour Government in 1997, a range of new policies has been put in place that aim to tackle social exclusion and improve the life chances of children and young people. The Government's approach spans a broad range of areas: education, social services, youth services and health services, as well as income support and employment, have all come under the spotlight. In this article we identify some of the factors that brought about the introduction of these policies and give an overview of some of the initiatives that have been introduced since 1997. We look at some of the key issues that will influence the implementation of these initiatives and also look at the contribution that young people can make to shaping local and national policy.

## CHILDREN: A NEW POLITICAL PRIORITY?

The *Independent Inquiry into Inequalities in Health*,[1] chaired by Sir Donald Acheson and commissioned by the then Minister of State for Public Health, Tessa Jowell, reiterated the findings of the 1980 Black Report,[2] which showed a strong link between health and economic status. Acheson's report, which promoted a socio-economic model of health, gave high priority to the health of families with young children, arguing that the interventions with the best chance of reducing future inequalities in mental and physical health were those that related to present and future mothers and children. Acheson's report, coming soon after government pledges to fight social exclusion and poverty, could not be ignored, and its influence is evident in some of the early cross-departmental policies such as Sure Start.

Over the course of Labour's first term in office, other factors have helped push children further up the political agenda. A series of high-profile cases of child abuse in children's homes, the recent case of Victoria (Anna) Climbie, in which the systematic abuse of an eight-year-old child went unnoticed by social workers, police and hospital staff, and the embarrassment of topping the European child poverty league tables, have contributed to a growing sense that public services do not support children and young people well.

In addition to concerns about the poor quality of public services for children, cost pressures and initiatives such as Best Value and Quality Protects in local government are giving additional impetus to central and local government to rethink the way public services for children are being delivered. A recent survey carried out by the Local Government Association showed that councils in England and Wales expect to overspend on social services for children by an estimated £128 million in the financial year 2000–01.

## GOVERNMENT RESPONSES

The Government's approach to tackling social exclusion and improving support for children and young people can be grouped in three broad categories: fiscal support and supply-side measures; targeted support for vulnerable children; and improving mainstream services, including education and health services.

### FISCAL SUPPORT AND SUPPLY-SIDE MEASURES

Under-18s have a powerful ally in the current Chancellor, Gordon Brown, who has been a strong advocate of fiscal measures to help meet the Government's target of abolishing child poverty within 20 years. Successive budgets have increased the level of child benefit by 25 per cent for the eldest child[3] and, reflecting the view that the best way to reduce child poverty is to get their parents into work and help them to stay there, a new working families tax credit and new assistance to cover some of the costs of child care have been introduced. Other supply-side measures such as the New Deal for Lone Parents have also helped to get parents of children at highest risk of poverty back into the labour market. For the Chancellor, this strategy is the key not only to reducing child poverty but also represents 'the best anti-drugs, anti-crime, anti-deprivation policy for our country'.[4] By the time of the 2001 election, estimates suggest that between 1.2 million and 1.5 million children may have been lifted out of poverty as a result of changes in the tax and benefit system and increases in the number of parents in work – still leaving around 3 million children in income poverty.[5]

### TARGETED SUPPORT FOR VULNERABLE CHILDREN

The second component of policy has been to target resources at particularly vulnerable children through the development of a wide range of area-based initiatives that aim to reduce poverty and social exclusion through local partnerships (see Box 1 overleaf). These include both schemes exclusively for children and their families such as Sure Start (led by the Department for Education and Skills (DfES)), which aims to deliver far-reaching impacts on the lives of children who pass through it by early intervention and support, and schemes with a broader community remit such as the Department of Transport, Local Government and the Regions' New Deal for Communities.

## BOX 1: TARGETED PROGRAMMES

**EARLY YEARS**

| | |
|---|---|
| Sure Start | 500 programmes by 2004 to promote the physical, intellectual and social development of children under 4 living in deprived areas |
| Sure Start Plus | 20 pilot schemes set up in March 2001 to support pregnant teenagers and teenage parents |

**COMMUNITY SAFETY**

| | |
|---|---|
| On Track | 24 projects in high-crime areas to work with children at risk of offending |

**HEALTH AND SOCIAL CARE**

| | |
|---|---|
| Health Action Zones | 26 areas designated to tackle health inequalities, working across local agencies. Most tackle the health of children and young people |

**EDUCATION AND TRAINING**

| | |
|---|---|
| Education Action Zones | Around £73 million to raise educational standards in areas of high deprivation |
| Excellence in Cities | Around £120 million per year to address educational problems in inner city schools through learning mentors and new specialist schools |

**REGENERATION AND SOCIAL EXCLUSION**

| | |
|---|---|
| New Deal for Communities | £800 million over three years to regenerate 39 of the most deprived parts of England by improving health and educational attainment and reducing crime and worklessness |

While it is still too early to evaluate the impact of many of these schemes, they indicate a welcome shift towards prevention, bringing together a wide range of different government departments working towards a common agenda and delivering against shared targets. This approach, piloted with Sure Start, is now being rolled out more widely in the wake of the report on young people by the Social Exclusion Unit's Policy Action Team, which highlighted the need for a more cohesive approach to the development and implementation of policy for young people.[6]

**REFORM OF MAINSTREAM SERVICES**

While the Government's approach initially focused on targeting the most vulnerable children, a second wave of policies aimed at reforming universal services for children and young people has also come under the spotlight (Box 2).

Included in this second wave is the NHS Plan, which sets out a number of measures to target children, including a wider role for midwives and improved screening programmes for women and children. In the pipeline is the national service framework for children and young

## BOX 2: REFORMS TO MAINSTREAM SERVICES

**EARLY YEARS**

National Childcare Strategy | £470 million strategy to provide good-quality child care to children up to the age of 14. Delivered through Early Years Development and Childcare Partnerships in every local authority area

**SOCIAL EXCLUSION**

Youth Offending Teams | Multi-agency teams, including representation from health, education, social services, police and probation services to reduce offending by young people

**HEALTH AND SOCIAL CARE**

Quality Protects | Universal reform of the management and delivery of children's social services (children looked after by local authorities, children in the child protection system and children with disabilities)

Healthy Schools Programme/ National Healthy School Standard | Schools to work with pupils to identify ways to develop health-promoting initiatives in schools

**EDUCATION AND TRAINING**

Connexions | £420 million to provide personal advisers appointed to all young people to give advice on careers, training and personal development

**REGENERATION & SOCIAL EXCLUSION**

Children's Fund | £450 million fund to support projects to prevent poverty and social exclusion for children aged 5 to 13

people, announced by the Secretary of State for Health in February 2001. Although the remit of this national service framework is still under discussion, it is likely to include national standards and service models for children's health and social services.

### ADDING IT ALL UP

Making sense of the wide range of initiatives put in place since 1997 to improve the life chances of children and young people, and co-ordinating the activities of the seven government departments that lead different children's programmes, will be the job of the newly established Children and Young People's Unit, which was set up on the recommendation of the Policy Action Team on Young People to give a national steer across government on children's services. This unit will have an important role, advising the Minister for Young People and a new cabinet committee on children and young people chaired by the Chancellor.

Crucial to the success of the unit will be its ability to coordinate a potentially baffling range of initiatives and new policies, and to come up with ways of bringing these together locally. Local mechanisms for children's services are complex, and the large number of planning processes involving a wide range of statutory and voluntary sector partners has made it difficult to create coherent local strategies.[7] The introduction of Local Strategic Partnerships (LSPs) in April 2001, bringing together different parts of the public sector with non-statutory organisations to co-ordinate the bewildering array of local plans and partnerships, has the potential to help close the gap between local services. Measures in the Health and Social Care Act to introduce Care Trusts, which would commission and provide integrated health and social services, also offer new opportunities to improve the integration of children's services.

## THE LONDON PICTURE

Within London, the pattern of services for children is beginning to shift at both strategic and operational level. Following the mayor's election commitment to make London a child-friendly city, work is going on to produce a Children's Strategy and to ensure that the mayor's statutory strategies around transport, development, bio-diversity, waste management, air quality, noise pollution, culture and spatial development reflect the needs and views of children. The mayor is being assisted in the development of this strategy by the newly formed Office of the Children's Rights Commissioner for London, working with a broad coalition of statutory and voluntary agencies.

While this strategy will need to focus on areas for which the mayor has formal responsibilities, it is important that strong links are maintained with other work underway in the capital, including strategic plans to improve children's health and social services that fall outside

the mayor's remit. A key ally will be the London Children's Taskforce, set up to oversee the implementation of the parts of the NHS Plan that relate to children but which will also be playing an important role in looking at ways to provide more 'joined-up' children's services in London.

## KEY QUESTIONS

While many of the new programmes that have been introduced do represent a significant shift in the services for children, there remain important questions about the impact this will have on mainstream health, education and social services for children. Many practitioners argue that the number of new initiatives and the speed with which they have been introduced have made it difficult to assess the impact of new forms of provision and suggest looking at ways that learning can be shared with colleagues.

Evidence from the evaluation of Health Action Zones (HAZs) has shown that, in some areas, mainstreaming innovative initiatives to promote health and well-being has been hampered by time constraints, organisational and cultural issues, and historic rivalries, particularly in areas with little history of previous partnership working.[8]

As partnership working becomes the norm for mainstream services providers, the learning from collaborative projects such as HAZs and Sure Start will need to inform the development of mainstream service provision. Staff will need to be equipped to understand – and feel comfortable working in – complex, fluid structures.

Evaluating the influence of new cross-sectoral initiatives on children's and young people's health and well-being is likely to be a major challenge. Although there is a large amount of literature supporting the link between social exclusion and health, there is little evidence about the impact of cross-sectoral schemes on health.[9] Disentangling the complex range of causal factors that act together to influence health and finding ways to analyse these factors in evaluation programmes will be an important challenge for researchers as new initiatives begin to take effect.

## CHILDREN KNOW BEST?

There is increasing recognition that young people have an important role to play in shaping and evaluating services. The UK is a signatory to the UN Convention on the Rights of the Child, which recognises children's fundamental rights to 'participation in the decisions that affect them and in the life of their community'. The Social Exclusion Unit's Policy Action Team on Young People identified the development of effective mechanisms for listening to children and

---

## BOX 3: INVOLVING YOUNG PEOPLE IN POLICY-MAKING AND SERVICE DELIVERY

CONSULTING YOUNG PEOPLE ON LOCAL SERVICES IN REDBRIDGE AND WALTHAM FOREST

Over the last five years, young people aged 11+ in Waltham Forest have shaped the development of *Face2Face*, to provide integrated health and social care in a range of community settings. Young people were given a say at different stages of service development using a range of methods:

- **Young people's priorities and how they should be met** – through a peer education health project with 72 young people on two social housing estates and a local school. Also, through participatory appraisal with 106 young people on another estate.
- **Ongoing service evaluation and development** – through routine data collection, focus groups and informal feedback.
- **Designing the service name and logo** – through a summer scheme run by the youth service.
- **Young People's Forum** – this is now being set up to ensure that young people continue to have a say in decision-making.

This needs-led approach to service development has united health and youth services with voluntary organisations to focus on young people's needs.

IMAGINE LONDON – INVOLVING YOUNG PEOPLE IN DECISIONS ABOUT HEALTH AND WELL-BEING IN LONDON

The King's Fund is working with young Londoners aged 11 to 18 to develop their ideas about ways to make London a healthier city, using a range of methods:

- young people-led events on transport, the environment, crime, healthy living and emotional well-being
- an interactive web site developed by young people (*www.imaginelondon.org.uk*)
- a youth assembly that will develop a young people's health manifesto for London.

young people as a key priority for government, a task that will now be implemented by the Children and Young People's Unit. This unit is in the process of setting up a young people's advisory forum to advise the Minister for Young People and to make sure that young people are central to the development of new policies. Within London, children's views will be at the core of the mayor's Children's Strategy, which will draw on the results of a recent consultation exercise[10] completed by around 3000 young people, and a number of other projects are underway locally to incorporate young people's views into service planning and delivery (Box 3).

## CONCLUSION

Evaluating the impact of the raft of policies to support children and young people will be a long-term process. Their success will depend on whether there is sufficient capacity at local level to work flexibly across organisational boundaries and to ensure that services reflect the needs and views of the young people who will be using them. Many of the early initiatives that have been put in place to develop more responsive local services offer useful lessons to help change the face of mainstream services. As new strategic plans are developed for London's children, these lessons will need to be absorbed.

## REFERENCES

1 Acheson D. *Independent inquiry into inequalities in health.* London: HMSO, 1998.
2 Black D et al. *Inequalities in health: report of a research working group.* London: DHSS, 1980.
3 Toynbee P, Walker D. *Did things get better? An audit of Labour's successes and failures.* London: Penguin Books, 2001.
4 Speech by the Chancellor of the Exchequer to the Children and Young People's Unit Conference at the Design Centre, Islington, London, on 15 November 2000.
5 Fimister G, editor. *An end in sight? Tackling child poverty in the UK.* London: Child Poverty Action Group, 2001.
6 National Strategy for Neighbourhood Renewal. *Report of Policy Action Team 12: young people.* London: Stationery Office, March 2000.
7 Department of Health. *Children's services planning consultation.* London: Department of Health, 2000. Available at *www.doh.gov.uk/scg/cspconsultation.htm*
8 Bauld L, Judge K, Lawson L, Mackenzie M, Mackinnon J, Truman J. *Health Action Zones in transition: progress in 2000.* Glasgow: University of Glasgow, 2000. Available at *www.haznet.org.uk*
9 Popay J, editor. *Regeneration and health: a selected review of research.* London: King's Fund and the Nuffield Institute for Health. Forthcoming.
10 *Sort it out! Children and young people's ideas for building a better London.* London: Office of the Children's Rights Commissioner for London, 2001.

# London emergency

Michael Damiani and Jennifer Dixon

There seems to be a crisis in the NHS each winter. The sudden increase in demand for hospital beds and NHS staff time is due to an increase in emergency admissions. The increased demand puts a huge strain on all parts of the NHS, especially acute hospitals, and significant shortcomings in NHS care frequently result, for example, in long waits for patients in A&E departments. Historically, efforts have been concentrated on finding ways to manage these peaks when they happen, rather than on finding a way to predict and, ultimately, to prevent their consequences on NHS care.

In the summer of 2000, the London Regional Office of the NHS Executive commissioned the King's Fund to analyse winter pressures on the NHS in London arising from emergency admissions. The objectives of the work included an investigation of the volume of emergency admissions over time, the reasons why patients were being admitted, and which groups of patients were being admitted most frequently.

The Hospital Episode Statistics (HES) for three years (1997/8 to 1999/2000) were acquired from the Department of Health. The HES data obtained included all 'finished consultant episodes' of London residents and patients registered with a general practice within the London NHS Region. Every record in the data set included a set of diagnostic codes, coded by the International Classification of Diseases, Injuries and Causes of Death, 10th revision (ICD–10). These codes can be grouped into 'chapters' and 'subchapters' of ICD–10, in which codes are grouped into broad diseases, such as respiratory disease or cancers. There are 20 chapters, defining categories of disease and other reasons for seeking medical attention. We present here initial analysis of these data.

The analysis revealed some interesting patterns. Looking at data for all emergency admissions, these varied only moderately from month to month. The pattern was similar for elective admissions (which mainly include non-emergency surgery). However, analysis of emergency admissions by month by broad illness type (by ICD–10, chapter 10) produced some interesting results (see Figure 1).

Figure 1 shows the total number of emergency admissions per week, by broad disease group across the London region as a whole. Data from the three-year period from 1 April 1997 to 31 March 2000 are shown.

# Figure 1: Weekly number of emergency admissions by ICD chapter

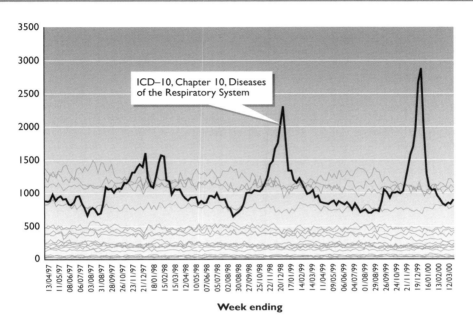

ICD–10, Chapter 10, Diseases of the Respiratory System

**Week ending**

For most disease groups, the total number of weekly emergency admissions did not vary a great deal over the three years. With the obvious exception of diseases of the respiratory system (ICD–10, chapter 10), there was only moderate seasonal variation. Admissions for respiratory disease represented approximately 13 per cent of the total number of emergency admissions in the period studied.

For this disease group there were clear peaks in the winter months, especially in late December and early January. An interesting phenomenon was the double peak in winter 1997/8 – first in December 1997 and then again in the second half of February 1998. This pattern is almost identical to that of the rates of GP consultations for influenza and influenza-like illness in England over the same time

period supplied by the Public Health Laboratory Service.

Additional analysis of the pattern of emergency admissions for respiratory disease further revealed that the seasonal variation observed could largely be attributed to diagnoses in six ICD subchapters: bronchiolitis, pneumonia, asthma, chronic obstructive airways disease (COAD), 'other' acute upper respiratory infections, and 'other' acute lower respiratory infections.

Age is a major factor that determines which of those six types of respiratory disease people are mostly affected by (see Figure 2).

Figure 2 shows the numbers of emergency admissions in each of the six ICD

## Figure 2: Main respiratory emergency admissions by age (all diagnostic codes)

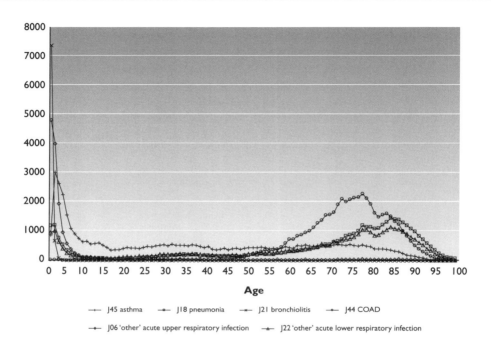

subchapters by age of admission, using data for all three study years. It can be seen that there was a peak in emergency admissions for bronchiolitis in children under two years of age, whereas admissions for acute upper respiratory infections peaked in children under about eight years of age. Admissions for three lower respiratory conditions – pneumonia, 'other' acute lower respiratory infection and chronic obstructive airways disease – occurred mainly in people aged 55 or over. On the other hand, admissions for asthma peaked in children aged one, declined rapidly until age 15, and then remained steady until old age. Emergency admissions for respiratory disease in older children and young adults were almost exclusively because of asthma.

Apart from asthma, emergency admissions of older adults with respiratory disease were mostly due to lower respiratory infections, especially after the age of about 55. Of these, the highest number of emergency admissions occurred in people with COAD, peaking at the age of 75 and declining thereafter, possibly due to the smaller number of people in older age groups.

Looking at seasonal variation, emergency admissions for all these broad groups of respiratory disease (except for asthma) peaked in winter. Again, this pattern was almost identical to the seasonal pattern in the rates of GP consultations for influenza and influenza-like illness obtained from the Public Health

Laboratory Service. It is noticeable that the number of emergency admissions in winter for influenza was very low (data not shown), which means either that admissions for influenza were not being coded accurately, GP consultations recorded as for influenza and influenza-like illness were in fact consultations for the respiratory diseases shown in the graph, or that influenza could trigger respiratory disease in the young and old, particularly in those prone to wheezing and asthma and in those with chronic respiratory disease. The number of emergency admissions for asthma appeared to peak in September every year rather than December.

Clearly, understanding the changes in the numbers of emergency admissions is vital for those responsible for managing NHS services in London over winter. However, the demands these admissions are likely to place on the health service, the extent of NHS resources the patients are likely to consume during the period of care, and which patients are likely to consume the most resources, is more relevant.

To help tackle these questions, we calculated the average length of stay of patients admitted with respiratory disease by age, and then the total number of bed days these patients occupied. Figure 3 shows the results, using data for all three study years combined.

Looking at the lowest line, the graph shows that the total number of emergency admissions for all respiratory

## Figure 3: Length of stay for respiratory emergencies by age

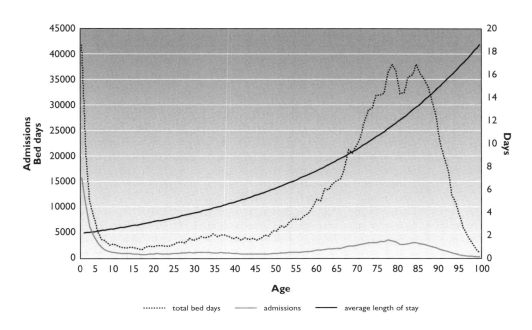

......... total bed days  ——— admissions  ——— average length of stay

diseases was high at age 0–5, then declined steeply to a low level before rising with age, as shown in Figure 2. The top line on the graph shows the average length of stay in hospital – that is, the number of bed days occupied divided by the number of admissions. This rose from about two days for children to over 16 days for very old people.

This graph indicates that the biggest demand on NHS resources (in terms of bed days) from patients with respiratory disease admitted as emergencies will occur in patients aged 55 and older. While Figure 2 shows that there was a high volume of emergency admissions in children under five with bronchiolitis and upper respiratory tract infection, 'winter pressures' on the NHS are more likely to arise from patients aged 55 and older, admitted with lower respiratory infection, particularly as a result of COAD.

Patients with COAD, since they have a chronic disease, are identifiable to the NHS in advance of having an acute episode of illness resulting in admission. Such patients will be known to their GPs, and may have a history of respiratory illness leading to hospital admission. Our rather simple analysis presented here strongly suggests that efforts to manage winter pressures should focus on these patients. Management of this group of patients should be proactive, should focus on primary care, and should occur well before patients become ill. This may mean ensuring that these patients are vaccinated against influenza, are monitored frequently during the winter months, and are treated at the earliest sign of infection. Furthermore, getting these patients home post-discharge from hospital should also be a priority, and hospitals should work particularly closely with social services staff specifically for this group of patients. Again, social services could be alerted and briefed in advance of illness for this particular group.

## ACKNOWLEDGEMENTS

We would like to thank Philip Brown and Chris Garrett at the NHS Executive, London Regional Office, and Sue Meehan and her colleagues at the London Ambulance Service for their help and support for this project. Funding: London Regional Office.

# Health and London governance

## Anna Coote and Ruth Tennant

### INTRODUCTION

Only four years ago, the place of health in London governance looked very different from the way it does today: the National Health Service was split between two London regional offices; there was no directly elected London-wide authority; there was no organisation – except, perhaps, for the King's Fund – that spoke for health and health care across the capital. Now that has all changed. But what do the new arrangements promise for the health of Londoners? We know that there are profound inequalities in health and health care. If you live in Tower Hamlets, you are twice as likely to die before you are 75 than if you live in Kingston upon Thames. Infant mortality rates are ten times higher in some London boroughs than in others. These alarming figures, which are just the tip of an iceberg, point to a need for a far more focused and co-ordinated approach to health than in the past.

In this paper we trace the emergence of a pan-London approach to health improvement through a series of steps, including the establishment of the London Health Commission. We outline the beginnings of a cross-sectoral strategy for London's health and describe the first health impact assessments of new pan-London initiatives, including strategies for London's transport and economic development. We consider the scrutiny powers of the London Assembly and explore the implications for London of devolution and emerging regionalism in the UK. Finally, we draw on international comparisons to see how other city-wide authorities have used whatever means they have at their disposal to improve health.

### TOWARDS A HEALTH STRATEGY FOR LONDON

The case for a London-wide health strategy was argued in 1997 by the King's Fund London Commission. Its report recommended a 'public health strategy for Londoners, building on community development initiatives that link local government and local health services in community regeneration and renewal of the urban fabric'. Londoners' 'growing health inequalities' should be a priority, the report said, and the strategy 'should take account of interactions between health services and other factors impacting on health, such as transport, housing, employment and environmental issues'.[1] More controversially, the Commission called for new public health responsibilities for the capital and specific functions for regulating health service provision to be created within the Government Office for London and later transferred to whatever 'new structures' were agreed for the capital.

A year later, in 1998, the first public health report for London was produced by the Health of Londoners Project (HOLP), funded by London health authorities. It recommended 'a clear pan-London dimension to London's health strategies'. This was needed, the report said:

- to help cope with London's particularly complex administrative structures
- to be able to define inequalities in health across the whole city to direct priorities for investment
- to develop a better comparative framework for monitoring health
- to tackle problems such as transport, air pollution and specialist drug treatment that could not be addressed effectively by individual health authorities
- to 'be able to develop a common framework for linking public health policy for London between the NHS, London government and other organisations'.[2]

In the same year, the Government produced the White Paper *A Mayor and Assembly for London*.[3] This proposed that 'The Mayor would look at the effect on health of all his or her policies and functions and would have a duty to promote the improvement of the health of Londoners'. It gave the Greater London Authority (GLA) no responsibility for health strategy in London, but the statutory duty to promote health improvement in London seemed to promise a positive engagement with the public health agenda. It came as a blow to some, therefore, when the GLA Bill, published in 1999, not only failed to give the new authority any responsibility for health strategy, but also omitted the duty to improve health. It merely said that in preparing and revising the strategies for which the new authority was to be responsible, it must 'have regard' to the desirability of 'promoting improvements in the health of persons in Greater London'.

A more positive development in the same year was the establishment of a single London Regional Office of the NHS Executive, anticipating the arrival of a London-wide elected authority and with coterminous boundaries. Dr Sue Atkinson was appointed as the first Director of Public Health to have responsibility for London as a whole.

There are probably three main reasons why the Bill retreated from the ground occupied by the White Paper. First, the NHS in London was reluctant to encourage any encroachment of the new London Authority on its domain. Fears were expressed at the time of a 'take-over by the mayor'. Any mention of health in the draft legislation was seen as a threat, opening the way to interference by elected regional government in running London's health services. Second, the London boroughs, anxious to protect their own territory, were inclined to resist anything that would enhance the power of the new authority, including a duty to improve health. Third, health had not yet registered on the radar system of the Government Office for London as a key factor in urban regeneration: they were preoccupied by the pressing demands of other sectors such as transport, economic development and environment. So, the leading government department was indifferent to health and the two sectors with most power to lobby for its inclusion had their own reasons for holding back. It was left to a handful of individuals and voluntary organisations to make the case for a stronger role in health for the new mayor.

The King's Fund, commenting on the shortcomings of the Bill, stressed that it was 'not arguing for the Mayor to have any executive powers over health services in London' but that 'the public health baby has been thrown out with the NHS bath water'. It proposed that the London Mayor should have a specific duty to promote the health of Londoners and to conduct health impact assessments of GLA policies. The Mayor should 'convene a London Health Improvement Forum, to include Assembly members, appointees from the London Region [of the NHS], from London boroughs and health authorities and other relevant agencies to promote a shared approach to planning for health across the capital'.[4]

## A LONDON-WIDE PARTNERSHIP FOR HEALTH

Early in 1999, the first practical steps were taken that would lead to the establishment of the London Health Commission. The London Region of the NHS took the initiative in forming a partnership of London organisations, including the Government Office for London, the Association for London Government, the Social Services Inspectorate and the King's Fund. On 19 May, a day-long conference entitled 'Towards a Health Strategy for London' attracted more than 400 people from across the capital. This set the pattern for the next year, which saw a series of inclusive, cross-sectoral events focusing on upstream determinants of health and inequalities, rather than on health services, and committed to developing a strong coalition with an action-oriented strategy in advance of the Mayor's election. A steering group was set up to pull together work plans and engage with Londoners 'as widely as possible in developing the outline framework' for a health strategy.

By the time the GLA Act had completed its course through Parliament in November 1999, it had been amended to give the new Authority a stronger role in health improvement. The Act sets out the 'principal purposes' of the GLA, which are to promote economic development and wealth creation, social development and improvement of the environment in Greater London. The Authority has 'power to do anything which it considers will further any one or more of its principal purposes'. In deciding whether or how to exercise such power, it must not only 'have regard to the effect ... on the health of persons in Greater London' but also 'do so in the way which it considers best calculated to promote improvements in the health of persons in Greater London'. The same measures are provided for 'the achievement of sustainable development in the United Kingdom'.[5] These subsidiary powers are limited however: the Authority need not do anything to promote health or sustainable development that is not 'reasonably practicable in all the circumstances of the case'. And it is explicitly barred from incurring expenditure in providing any housing, education, social service or health service.

In December 1999, more than 450 people attended a second conference, described by Dr Atkinson as a 'staging post in a dynamic development process' intended to produce 'a strategy which we can share with the Mayor and the Greater London Authority'.[6] By now, the NHS in London was less anxious about encroachments by the Mayor. It was widely thought at the time that the former Health Secretary and preferred candidate of Downing Street, Frank Dobson, would win the election. Had the prospect of Ken Livingstone storming to victory been more apparent, the mood might have been more jumpy, for Livingstone was often heard to say that he thought the new London Authority should – in the long run – be responsible for London's health services.

But another factor was causing the retentiveness of 1998/9 to loosen. The London Health Strategy Group was growing into a strong cross-sectoral alliance that was increasingly confident and enthusiastic about a pan-London approach to health improvement. Its members represented, in addition to the founding partners, some individual boroughs and health authorities, a range of voluntary organisations, embryonic functional bodies of the GLA (including those concerned with transport and economic development) and other key players such as the pro-business group London First, Social Enterprise London and London Borough Grants. Most were genuinely taken with the idea of a partnership to promote the health of Londoners and (since most came from outside the NHS) they had no difficulty in distinguishing an initiative to tackle the causes of ill health from one that aimed to improve or appropriate health services. So, there was a clear agenda that did not threaten the NHS or marginalise the boroughs and that manifestly needed to include business and the 'third sector'. There had never been such a partnership before, so the experience was fresh and invigorating. It was evident by early 2000 that the best way to meet whatever challenges might issue from the newly elected Authority was to firm up the group and draw up a draft strategy that could be presented to the Mayor as a *fait accompli*.

March 2000 saw the launch of an 'Outline Strategic Framework' for a

London Health Strategy,[7] which, among other things, established a London Coalition for Health and Regeneration, based on the original strategy group. The accompanying literature[8] said that 'a thousand people from more than 300 organisations' had worked on the strategy and had 'identified four priority areas for action: regeneration, inequalities, Black and minority ethnic health and transport'. It announced plans to set up a London Health Observatory (in line with government policy to have one in every region) that would 'bring together the information and expertise needed to analyse, research and report on health across the capital'. There were plans on each of the priority areas that needed 'to be developed into deliverable actions' – for example, to ensure that London's regeneration programmes included an emphasis on health improvement, to improve advice and access to benefits for poor Londoners, and to develop shared programmes to tackle institutional racism, and methods to assess the impact of transport policies on health. The London Health Observatory would 'develop the high level health indicators which have been identified under the health strategy into a monitoring programme'. The said indicators included rates of overall and minority ethnic unemployment, GCSE attainment, unfit housing, burglary, poor air quality, traffic accidents, life expectancy, infant deaths and self-reported fair, poor or bad health.

## ENTER THE MAYOR AND THE COMMISSION

In May 2000, Ken Livingstone was elected Mayor of London, in spite of concerted efforts by the Prime Minister and New Labour to win votes for 'their' man. Jeffrey Archer, who at one point looked a formidable contender, had fallen from grace. Stephen Norris, who then became the Tory candidate, seemed to impress London's elites more than the bulk of voters. The Green Party's Darren Johnson and the Liberal Democrats' Susan Kramer were never serious challengers. Glenda Jackson lacked any real base in London. And poor Frank Dobson found that his greatest asset – energetic backing from Downing Street – was also his greatest liability. All the main candidates had included health as a significant element in their manifestos, a sign that the emerging Coalition on Health and Regeneration had succeeded in moving the issue up London's political agenda. Livingstone pledged to establish a London Health Commission with a broad-based membership that would advise the Mayor, with particular reference to tackling inequalities, ensuring sustainability of initiatives, and promoting the health of Londoners.

If Livingstone's victory came as a surprise to some, so did the assiduous diplomacy with which he handled his accession. On the health front, he appointed Dr Atkinson to his advisory cabinet. He fell silent on the issue of who should control London's NHS. He welcomed the Coalition with its Outline Strategic Framework as the basis on which to build the Health Commission. He appointed Ansel Wong as chair, and his equalities adviser, Lee Jasper, as a member, and insisted – quite appropriately – on increasing the representation of black and minority ethnic groups. He accepted that the Commission would be independent, rather than under direct mayoral control. It all added up to a peaceful transition that pleased most of the participants, enabling them to focus on developing the strategy rather than on the political in-fighting that many had feared would follow the election.

The first meeting of the London Health Commission was on 12 October 2000, with the Mayor in attendance. The Commission's terms of reference were to develop, drive and monitor the London Health Strategy, to consider and advise on the health dimensions of key London-wide strategies, to promote health improvement and the reduction of inequalities, and to initiate and manage any action to promote the work of the Commission and the aims of the health strategy. In addition, members committed themselves to a set of core principles: actively involving citizens and communities; working in partnership; expanding and sharing intelligence on health and related issues; and working for equity at every level.

## ASSESSING THE MAYORAL STRATEGIES

The report On the Move,[9] which set out evidence of links between transport and health, was launched at the inaugural meeting. This was the first step in a health impact assessment (HIA) of the draft strategy for London's transport. The GLA had been charged with producing strategies for transport, economic development, bio-diversity, air quality, spatial development, culture, waste and noise, and had pledged to produce one on energy as well. Over the following months, the Health Commission's time was largely taken up with conducting health impact assessments, as draft mayoral strategies hit the table at an energetic pace. Within six months, the Commission had completed four HIAs – on transport, economic development, bio-diversity and air quality. Each one followed approximately the same procedure. First, a review of the literature was conducted to identify evidence of links between health and the subject of the strategy. Second, a rapid appraisal workshop was held, in which a wide range of 'stakeholders' reviewed the evidence and the strategy in the light of their own experience and expertise. Third, the conclusions of the workshop were considered by the whole Commission. Finally, the assessment was distilled into a report, with recommendations to the relevant strategic body. In each case, the approach was collaborative rather than confrontational, with the strategic body ostensibly welcoming the assessment and participating in it.

It is hard to gauge how influential these HIAs have been. At the time of writing, only one strategy – that on transport – had received the Commission's recommendations and produced a final strategy for consultation. The recommendations had included proposals to promote cycling and walking, to segregate modes of transport by reallocating routes, and to link congestion charging with emissions and with low-emission zones. A paper presented to the Commission in January 2001, which attempted to assess the impact of the HIA, claimed that many of the recommendations had been adopted, but not the one relating to congestion charging. *The Mayor's Transport Strategy*, which runs to 331 pages, acknowledges the work of the London Health Commission and the important role transport can play in damaging and improving health.[10]

The HIA on the GLA's draft Economic Development Strategy was led by the King's Fund and completed in March 2001. Among its recommendations were:

- to make health improvement a key policy objective
- to include health outcomes as success criteria for regeneration

- to consider requiring projects funded by the London Development Agency to carry out HIAs on their plans and programmes
- to acknowledge the crucial role in regeneration played by the NHS as an employer and contractor
- to invite the NHS and local authorities to be key signatories to the Strategy.

It remains to be seen how far these are taken up by the LDA.

It became clear in the course of these early HIAs that evidence linking health to mayoral strategies was thin on the ground. Producing an evidence-based case for amending any of them in the interests of health was seldom an option. The HIA process was therefore less about 'scientifically' proving that one course of action or another was good or bad for health, and more about advocating health improvement and raising awareness among experts and stakeholders about the potential links with health.

Strikingly, the bulk of the Commission's HIA recommendations have had little to do with what are conventionally understood as 'health issues'. On the bio-diversity strategy, for example, it recommended working 'with the voluntary sector and other partners to address the key barriers people face in accessing green spaces, such as poor public transport links and perceived safety risks'. On air quality, the Commission urged, *inter alia*, an examination of 'how to capture the benefits which flow from reducing levels of traffic (e.g. reduced community severance, increased levels of exercise)' and a recognition that '"technical fixes" to air pollution will have more limited effects'. Proposals such as these reflected the Commission's broad definition of health and its focus on upstream determinants, which enabled it to see health improvement as a core function of all the GLA's strategic bodies. The latter were expected to operate within a policy framework that aimed not only to make London a world-class city, but also to reduce inequalities and improve the quality of life of Londoners. One aim of an HIA was, of course, to identify avoidable risks to health, but another – no less important – was to optimise benefits to health, and this was best achieved by helping to make each of the strategies more effective in its own terms.

## PRIORITIES FOR ACTION

The need to conduct health impact assessments dominated the Commission's agenda in its first six months. But by the summer of 2001, it was able to turn its attention to its own priorities for action (regeneration, inequalities, transport, and black and minority ethnic health). Sub-groups had been set up to develop and deliver work programmes on each of these. Early outputs included a health and regeneration learning network, consisting of 20 practitioners drawn from both sectors. A draft action plan for the Inequalities Priority Area, presented to the Commission in May 2001, set out three practical objectives: to develop a common framework for monitoring inequalities; to integrate strategies tackling inequalities at a local level; and to promote community involvement in strategies to tackle inequalities. The London Health Observatory, meanwhile, was mapping progress in London towards the new national health inequalities targets, and developing indicators to monitor the impact of the London Health Strategy.

As well as pursuing its own priorities, the Commission was expected to take an interest in other London-wide initiatives with implications for health, including the development of strategies on domestic violence, on alcohol and drugs, and for children. Its agenda was almost infinite, but its resources were not. In April 2001, there were 44 commissioners, supported by a very small secretariat made up of secondees from other organisations, accommodation was courtesy of the GLA, and there was modest *ad hoc* financial assistance from some of the sponsoring partners.

## CHALLENGES FOR THE FUTURE

An 'Action Evaluation of the London Health Commission' was carried out between January and April 2001 by independent consultants.[11] The subsequent (rather bland) report, based on interviews with 24 individuals and observations of meetings, found high levels of goodwill for the Commission and enthusiasm about its potential. It suggested that the Commission needed to be more widely known, more strongly linked to local partnerships, and more representative, especially of black and minority ethnic groups, schools and young people. The Commission could build on its stock of goodwill, said the report, by firming up its criteria for selecting 'workstreams' and identifying 'dedicated resources and support'.

As it moved towards its second year, the Commission could legitimately claim to be an inclusive partnership, backed by the Mayor, making its mark on the development of GLA policy and raising awareness – in elite circles if not among Londoners in general – about health and its determinants, about health inequalities in London, and about opportunities for health improvement through cross-sectoral working. It had scored some hits with its health impact assessments – and it had done all this on a shoestring, with goodwill as its major resource. It faced some formidable challenges: how to justify its existence by adding value to health-related work already underway across the capital; how to focus its activities and produce clear and creditable results; how to secure sufficient resources to enable it to be effective in the medium term; and how to communicate its messages to a wide range of Londoners, including senior policy-makers and opinion formers, practitioners, community leaders and hard-to-reach groups.

## PARALLEL ACTIVITIES

For all the challenges it faced, the London Health Commission at least had the advantage of a status and remit that was broadly understood and uncontested. Matters were not so clear within the GLA itself. The Authority's executive function is entirely in the hands of the Mayor. The Assembly, a 25-strong elected body, has oversight of key appointments and a modest budget, but no executive powers.

However, it does have important scrutiny powers. These enable it to examine, either through its committees or through the full Assembly, any matters that it considers to be of importance to Greater London. How health scrutiny will be divided up between the full Assembly and its committees is not yet clear. However, in its first year of operation, one committee in particular has taken a strong lead over health issues. The Environment and Sustainability Committee, chaired by Labour's Samantha Heath, set up a sub-group to

select health issues for scrutiny and identified four themes: smoking in public places, safe routes to schools, environmental improvements for pedestrians and the environmental impact of the NHS in London.

At the same time, the first chair of the Assembly, Trevor Phillips, the former television journalist who had once been tipped as Labour's mayoral candidate, declared a special interest in health policy. He also sat on the Environment and Sustainability Committee, and had been appointed chair of the London Inequalities and Public Health Task Force by the London Region of the NHS. Livingstone had appointed many prominent Assembly members to his cabinet, including Nicky Gavron, who became Deputy Mayor, but not Phillips, who was excluded by virtue of his position (in the first year) as chair of the Assembly.

In May 2001, the Mayor issued his first annual report, which reviewed activities in the GLA's first year and set out activities for 2001.[12] This announced that the GLA would be carrying out a review of health as part of its Best Value Programme, under which it must demonstrate that all the services delivered by the GLA group offer value for money, continue to improve each year and are developed in a way that is sustainable over time. The scope of this review, scheduled to be carried out in 2002/03, is not yet clear, but will include all activities carried out by the GLA 'family' that could have an impact on health.

Throughout the first year of the Authority's life, the relationship between the Mayor and the Assembly could best be described as in a state of flux. Should they be working closely together or at arms' length? If they shared the same objectives, should they pool resources – for example, to support the London Health Commission? (Assembly funds had been used to pay for research contributing to its health impact assessments.) Or should the Assembly maintain a distance so that it could exercise its scrutiny function objectively? How should the scrutiny function be divided between the Assembly and individual committees? And how should the GLA's Best Value responsibilities fit with its scrutiny function? Inevitably, these dilemmas were not just technical ones, but were shaped by the personalities involved and the relationships between them, as well as by the shifting uncertainties (some would say chaos) that were among the birth pangs of a new democratic organisation. It was clear from the outset that the way in which the Authority conducted its business would be built on convention as much as on the letter of the law, and that habits formed in the early months and years could exert a profound influence over its working patterns, culture and effectiveness in the longer term. Clarity of purpose and procedure would make it easier to build a strong role for the Authority in promoting the health of Londoners. Continuing uncertainties and interpersonal rivalries could have the opposite effect.

## DEVOLUTION AND THE GLA

Just as the development of internal conventions would affect the GLA in the medium to long term, so would trends towards increased local accountability and control across the UK. Evidence from other countries shows that regional governments often develop their powers incrementally, starting with a series of

basic functions that may be added to over time.[13] This dynamic is already visible in England, where the Government has signalled a commitment to increase the powers of Regional Development Agencies and regional chambers – made up of representatives of local government and social and economic partners – by moving towards directly elected regional government, where there is a will locally to do so.[14]

Mayor Livingstone has indicated that he will argue for greater powers for the GLA once discussions about the potential roles and responsibilities for regional government start to pick up speed. Notwithstanding his diplomatic silence on who should run the NHS, there remains speculation that he may try to negotiate additional responsibilities in this area.[15] Similar pressure may come from within the Assembly, where Trevor Phillips (who became deputy chair in May 2001) announced a review of the Authority's powers and functions one year after the GLA came into being.

Formal responsibilities for health services are, however, unlikely to be handed over either to the GLA or to elected regional chambers. Even John Prescott, the Government's staunchest advocate of regional government, seems to favour the idea of 'light touch' assemblies, taking the view that a pragmatic, incremental development will meet less resistance than a sudden introduction of powerful regional bodies. This points towards an asymmetrical approach to development, with some regional assemblies moving faster than others and acting as 'test grounds' for more sceptical parts of the country.

Even without formal responsibilities, Regional Development Agencies are already beginning to play an informal role in influencing local health services.[16] The North West RDA's economic development strategy recognised that a healthier population should be a specific by-product of the RDA's work in stimulating economic development, and that improvements in health would, in turn, help improve productivity. Three RDAs have referred to the contribution that health services themselves can make to economic development as employers and in the way they procure goods and services and locate their activities. Early work carried out by the King's Fund into the links between the NHS and regeneration suggests that, while useful connections are being made in some areas, the effects are patchy and the lessons need to be more widely applied.[17] Within London, the GLA has begun to pick up some of these messages: the London Health Commission is focusing on regeneration and has helped to influence, through its health impact assessment, the first economic development strategy of the London Development Agency.

## SHIFTING STRUCTURES IN THE NHS

There are some signs that the NHS would welcome closer collaboration with regional and local authorities. Work carried out by the Constitution Unit at University College London[18] showed that many of the major health issues identified by NHS regional offices addressed the social, economic and environmental determinants of health (such as transport and warmer housing) and fell beyond the usual remit of the NHS. There was some interest, the research suggested, in integrating NHS activities with local and regional organisations that carried responsibility for sub-national economic development.

This dynamic could be given extra impetus by changes in the organisation of the NHS. Regional offices are to be abolished in 2003 and replaced by regional directors for health and social care as part of a move towards greater decentralisation of health services through primary care trusts. Announcing the changes to health service structures, Secretary of State for Health Alan Milburn said that the new directors would be co-located within Government Offices for the Regions. This, he said, would help improve joint working between health, transport, regeneration and the environment, so that 'if new regional government structures emerge there will be a ready-made relationship with the NHS'.[19] Given the GLA's remit for many of the policy areas outlined by the Secretary of State, co-locating the relevant regional director within the GLA could be an important step towards strengthening the growing links between London government and the NHS. However, it is not clear how far the functions of the Government Offices for the Regions, which take orders directly from Whitehall, would ever be ceded to elected authorities, in London or anywhere else. A case in point is regeneration, where concerns over the growing powers of Regional Development Agencies have resulted in responsibilities for the financing and running of different regeneration programmes being split between national government (the Neighbourhood Renewal Unit), Government Offices for the Regions, and Regional Development Agencies. This suggests a certain reluctance to devolve further powers to the Regions.

## EXAMPLES FROM ACROSS THE UK

The Scottish and Welsh Assemblies have far greater power than the GLA, carrying as they do responsibility for the NHS, education and social services. There are, however, similarities between London and the two devolved administrations: Wales and Scotland have been described as 'policy villages', areas whose relatively small size makes it possible to experiment with cross-sectoral policies, a principle that could apply equally well to London.

*Better Wales*, the principal strategic document for the Welsh Assembly, included health improvement and the reduction of inequalities as one of its five priorities. This was outlined in more detail in the Assembly's consultation document *Promoting Health and Wellbeing*,[20] which stressed the importance of effective joint working between the Assembly, local councils, health services, voluntary organisations and local businesses in tackling the underlying causes of ill health. It urged all sectors to think of ways to 'build a better health dimension to the services they provide for the people and the communities they serve'. This covered a broad range of policy areas, including economic development, community planning, environmental and transport policies, and culture.

While the approach taken in London shares certain characteristics with that of the Welsh Assembly – both, for example, are conducting health impact assessments of major strategies – there are shades of difference. In Wales, health improvement has been mainstreamed into the Assembly's work and it is explicitly recognised that health cuts across all policy areas.[21] As *Better Wales* points out, the impact of its policies will not be evident in the short term. The Welsh example offers an important case study in developing effective multi-agency partnerships to improve health.

## THE DEMOCRATIC IMPERATIVE

One of the arguments that has been used in both Scotland and Wales to support the devolution of health services has been the need to make health services more locally accountable. Within Scotland, the Minister for Health and Community Care, Susan Deacon, has declared that 'Local communities and local people have a right to know who takes decisions and why they are taken and must have the opportunity to contribute to the decision-making process.'[22]

Local councils' newly acquired powers of scrutiny over local health services are a step towards increasing the democratic accountability in health policy at a local level. The Health and Social Care Act will allow them to review and scrutinise the operation of the health service in their area through overview and scrutiny committees (OSCs). It also requires health authorities to consult OSCs on major service changes. Chief executives of all NHS bodies will be required to appear before OSCs twice a year, and councils will be able to carry out scrutinies jointly with one or more neighbouring boroughs.

Although the GLA is not covered by the Health and Social Care Act, the Mayor could choose to use the good relations he has developed with the London Regional Office to promote local accountability for health services. The first two People's Question Times, held by the Mayor and Assembly, have already shown that Londoners have an appetite for asking questions about London's health. So far the Mayor has taken a diplomatic line on these questions, choosing not to get involved in headlong clashes with the NHS. But he has pointed out the need for working closely with the NHS to improve health and reduce inequalities. In future, the Mayor might want to invite his health adviser or another representative of the London Regional Office to attend his Question Time to demonstrate that the two organisations are working together and to help open up the NHS to public scrutiny.

## LEARNING FROM ELSEWHERE

As we have noted, the first year of the GLA has been a time of transition and change. Recruiting staff and learning how to work in a new organisation has inevitably taken time and there has been little opportunity to step back from day-to-day business and assess what impact the new body has had on London or to look for ideas from beyond the capital. However, there are signs that the GLA is building alliances beyond London, particularly with international cities that have common characteristics. Mayor Livingstone has created strong links with New York and is setting up friendship agreements with a range of cities across the world.

Work carried out by the King's Fund[23] suggests that such international links can offer useful insights into changing patterns of political power and influence in local government. Within the US, for example, city authorities have been a dynamic source of new ideas over the past decade, with a new cohort of mayors who have emerged as powerful political entrepreneurs.[24] These mayors may act as useful role models for aspiring political leaders in UK cities such as Manchester, Leeds, Glasgow and Cardiff, which are often described as experiencing a 'renaissance'.

International links can also shed light on ways to integrate health improving goals in mainstream policies. In Rome, former Mayor Francesco Rutelli made the reduction of accidents and rates of respiratory conditions a central part of his transport reforms, which have cut back traffic levels in the centre of Rome, introduced cleaner forms of public transport and brought in subsidies for scooters and cycle helmets. This type of intervention may be the most effective way of influencing some of the upstream determinants, such as environmental pollution, housing and employment, that have an important impact on people's underlying health status.

The strategic overview of a mayor can help to shine a spotlight on areas of the city in greatest need through effective use of city-wide data. In New York, Mayor Rudy Giuliani introduced Compstat – a detailed package of statistics on crime rates across the city that was used to track crime trends and to hold city police commanders to account. This technique has been widely copied elsewhere in the US, and the Mayor of Baltimore, Martin O'Malley, has adopted the technique to cover all aspects of the city's administration, ranging from lead poisoning and youth crimes to drug treatment centres.

## CONCLUSIONS

It is reasonable to speculate that recent developments in the UK could lead, eventually, to the GLA playing a more significant part in health improvement and health care, including the NHS. In general, however, the GLA has more limited powers and responsibilities than any comparable city-wide authority and, where health is concerned, its formal remit is negligible. However, the King's Fund's research into the experiences of other cities suggests that the personality of the Mayor and political context in which he or she operates are more likely to determine whether action is taken to improve health, than are formal powers and institutional arrangements. He or she is 'more likely to take action to improve health if it fits in with plans to pursue other major political objectives'. And a mayor with few direct powers can nevertheless contribute to health improvement 'through political influence, media campaigning, financial leverage and other, indirect means'.[25]

What has happened in London since the arrival of the Greater London Authority seems to bear out this point. Whether future health policies are developed more or less effectively, whether partnerships are stronger or weaker, whether or not strategies are implemented that begin to reduce health inequalities across the capital, may owe as much to informal politics, with a small 'p', and even to chance, as to the letter of the law or the stated intentions of government.

We asked at the outset what the new arrangements promise for the health of Londoners. Health is now firmly on the agenda of the GLA, which has the capacity, at least, to influence health policy and, at most, to promote the active pursuit of strategies to reduce health inequalities across the capital. In addition, there is an increasingly close partnership between a single London regional office of the NHS and the GLA, with the London Health Commission bringing together a wide range of London organisations in a cross-sectoral partnership committed to health improvement. Does this augur well? It is too early to reach a definitive view, but the current conditions appear to be more favourable to London's health than those prevailing before 1999.

## REFERENCES

1 King's Fund London Commission. *Transforming health in London*. London: King's Fund, 1997. p 132.

2 Health of Londoners Project. *The health of Londoners*. London: King's Fund, 1998. p xix.

3 Department of Environment, Transport and the Regions. *A mayor and assembly for London*. Cm 3897. London: The Stationery Office, 1998.

4 Davies A, Kendall E. *Health and the London mayor*. London: King's Fund, 1999. p 2.

5 Davies A, Kendall E. *Improving London's health: the role of the Greater London Authority*. London: King's Fund, 2000. p 6.

6 NHS Executive London Regional Office. 'London's Health' series, February 2000. *Moving forward. www.londonshealth.gov.uk*

7 NHS Executive London Regional Office. 'London's Health' series, March 2000. *The London Health Strategy: outline strategic framework. www.londonshealth.gov.uk*

8 NHS Executive London Regional Office. 'London's Health' series, March 2000. *A coalition for health and regeneration. www.londonshealth.gov.uk*

9 NHS Executive London Regional Office. 'London's Health' series, October 2000. *On the move. www.londonshealth.gov.uk*

10 Greater London Authority. *The mayor's transport strategy*. London: GLA, 2001. pp 26–8.

11 Mann Weaver. *Action based evaluation of the London Health Commission*, unpublished paper, May 2001.

12 Greater London Authority. *Annual Report 2001*. London: GLA, 2001. p 39. *www.london.gov.uk*

13 Russell Barter W. *Regional government in England: a preliminary review of literature and research findings*. London: Local and Regional Government Research Unit, DETR, October 2000.

14 1997 Labour Party manifesto.

15 Mayor seeks to build on record of achievements. *Financial Times* 2001; 3 May.

16 Jervis P, Plowden W, editors. *Devolution and health: first annual report of a project to monitor the impact of devolution on the United Kingdom's health services*. London: The Constitution Unit, 2000. *www.ucl.ac.uk/constitutionunit/d&h/index.htm*

17 *Health and regeneration: programme summary*. King's Fund briefing. London: King's Fund, 2000.

18 Jervis P, Plowden W, editors. *Op. cit.*, p 72.

19 Shifting the balance of power in the NHS. Speech by Alan Milburn, Secretary of State for Health, delivered on 25 April 2001. *http://tap.ccta.gov.uk/doh/interpress.nsf/page/2001-0200*

20 National Assembly for Wales. *Promoting health and wellbeing: implementing the national health promotion strategy*. Cardiff: National Assembly for Wales, 2000.

21 National Assembly for Wales. *Developing health impact assessment in Wales*. Cardiff: National Assembly for Wales, 2000.

22 Jervis P, Plowden W, editors. *Op. cit.*, p 88.

23 Davies A, Kendall E. *Op. cit.*, p 82.

24 Clark J, Hambleton R. *Models of local government: a transatlantic policy exchange. Briefing paper on US local government*. UK/US Centre for Local Government: 1999.

25 Davies A, Kendall E. *Op. cit.*, p 82.

# Community safety

## David Woodhead

### INTRODUCTION

'Community safety' is an umbrella term that draws together a range of issues affecting the safety and well-being of individuals and communities. It entails consideration of safety issues broadly, including fire, falls and accidents, access to safe green spaces, and good urban design. In addition, community safety activities focus on the causes and effects of burglary, violence, sex and hate crimes, and crimes related to the misuse of drugs and other substances. It is also concerned with ending 'sub-criminal' and anti-social behaviours, such as truancy, noise pollution and vandalism. When seen in these terms, the connections with the public health agenda are clear. The WHO definition of health – as 'a state of complete physical, mental and social wellbeing, and not merely the absence of disease or infirmity' – demonstrates the conceptual synergies. What makes a 'healthy community' is similar to what makes a safe one. Holistic views underpin both. Just as 'health' is not simply the absence of disease, a 'safe community' is not simply one with an absence of crime.

To investigate the health impacts of community safety, the role of health services in improving community safety, and the NHS as a provider of services for those affected by poor community safety (for example, victims of crime), early in 2001 the King's Fund interviewed around 40 public and voluntary sector policy-makers, managers and practitioners in London.

The study analysed the opinions of individuals working at the interface of health and community safety issues – including health services, local authorities and voluntary sector agencies, as well as other associated organisations including the police, probation service, prisons and the civil service. While it has provided a snapshot of views expressed in London on community safety issues, further research is needed to validate the findings and to provide a fuller picture. Questions were asked about 'community safety and health' in broad terms. However, what emerged from respondents' answers was a serious concern about crime and its impact on health.

### HEALTH AND COMMUNITY SAFETY – EXPLORING THE CONNECTIONS

Respondents spoke at length about recent mapping of criminal activity that has identified local 'hot spots' – areas where theft, violence and drug-related crimes are high. They pointed out that these hot spots often corresponded to identified areas of high morbidity and mortality as well as low income and general exclusion. As one local authority officer noted: 'Risk factors for poor health coincide with the risk factors for patterns and prevalence of crime.' Another pointed out that 'any community with a high score on Jarman (a composite indicator of socio-economic deprivation) is going to be an area of high crime'. For many, these corresponding factors suggested a relationship between poverty, social exclusion, poor health and high crime rates. Issues of community safety and its relation to health were, on the whole, issues of social inequality. Several respondents pointed to the disproportionate involvement of certain groups as victims and perpetrators of crime: vulnerable young people (including 'children looked after'), people with low educational achievement, people with severe and enduring mental illness, homeless people, and people from black and minority ethnic communities. They took the view that criminal activity, as with many complex health issues, could be both a cause and a result of social exclusion.

The realities and perceptions of crime were seen to have considerable effects on the mental and physical health of Londoners. Many respondents argued that poor levels of community safety made people ill. They stressed that the picture was complex and solutions would not be found by organisations working in isolation. The effects of poor community safety on health varied across time and space. Generally, it was agreed that poor community safety affected health, but as one respondent noted: 'The linkages remain poorly defined … especially where it is difficult to measure in concrete terms.'

However, there was general agreement that community safety and health *were* related in many ways. First, there were discernible physical effects, including injury from attack, from being hit by cars, or from fire:

> Children in social class V are 15 times more likely to die in a house fire than children in social class I, and kids living in temporary accommodation are up to 70 times more likely to die in fires. With evidence so stark, we should be doing something and doing it soon.

Second, there were diverse effects on individuals' mental health and sense of well-being. Third, several respondents pointed out that poor mental health could result in poor physical health over long periods of time (for example, digestion problems, skin conditions and hair loss). This was especially true for people living in poor environments over long periods of time, or for people who were repeatedly victimised.

The characteristics of areas where crimes were committed and experienced were a strong theme for the respondents. Street crime and the presence of street drinkers and drug dealers were thought to affect individuals' feelings of safety and sense of well-being. Drug dealing along certain streets allegedly stopped individuals, especially older people, from shopping there, occasionally barring access to food. Equally, crime could stop individuals walking in parks, making physical activity difficult.

Fear of crime featured prominently. Respondents argued that fear affected individuals' self-confidence and could alter their use of public facilities and public spaces. According to one health strategist: 'Sometimes, their perceptions do not correspond to reality.' Nevertheless, fears were acute:

> The way people see the situation can be very different from the reality; women are a great deal safer on trains than they are in their own homes … whereas young men are more likely to be attacked in public and are better off staying at home. This contradicts what we often think is true.

The gap between perception and reality posed a particular challenge. As a consultant in public health medicine claimed: 'The fear of crime imprisons older people; they often feel incapable of leaving their homes.' This theme recurred throughout our interviews. As one community representative noted: 'The old people on the estate do not believe that they can walk out of their front doors, go to the shops without feeling in danger of being mugged or shouted at or asked for money.' Fear of crime reduced the amount of exercise they could take and stopped them from seeing their families and friends. It affected their mental health and well-being, and was seen as a poorly researched area. In particular, hate crimes, including racist, homophobic and domestic violence, were thought to deserve greater attention, as were safety issues for disabled people. Racist crime was isolating: it stopped people from going out into the street. Respondents observed that too little was known about the effects of violence on the health and well-being of refugees and asylum seekers. Specialist services, for example drug rehabilitation, were often inaccessible to black and ethnic minority people.

Crimes against gay men and lesbians might go unreported because of fears of being treated unfairly by statutory services, several respondents revealed. 'There are still some gay men and lesbians who believe that they will be treated badly, that they live in a deeply homophobic society,' one voluntary sector respondent noted. Others claimed that individuals who had been attacked for being gay might attend A&E departments but decide not to cite the reason for the injury.

Victims of domestic violence were often left unsupported and felt unable to talk about their experiences until several years into a history of abuse. As one respondent from the voluntary sector noted:

'Domestic violence is more common than people think.' In particular, it was noted, especially with regard to domestic violence, that repeat victimisation had cumulative negative effects on health. The coupling of physical effects with long-term consequences for mental health was considered to be a particular challenge for health services. However, unlike other community safety issues, domestic violence was experienced across all social classes and was not directly associated with poverty and deprivation.

Violence against women was discussed at length by many of our interviewees. One noted that it should be recognised as a specific category of crime: 'Women are more likely to be attacked, to experience sexual assault, rape and harassment. It is an issue of gender and should be a priority.' Violence experienced and witnessed by children and young people was thought to cause and contribute to trauma, exclusion and renewed patterns of violence, as well as threatening educational attainment in the long term. One respondent commented: 'And so they grow up to be unemployed, poor, excluded, and unhealthy, just as their parents are.'

## THE ROLE OF THE NHS

All our respondents said that the NHS could be doing more to alleviate the effects of crime, although several noted that there were areas where the health sector had taken a strong role, for example in Crime and Disorder partnerships in Southwark. Three main areas were identified where the health service could do more to improve its performance.

First, it should take an active role in local regeneration initiatives that had strong community safety elements. This would help tackle the upstream determinants of health and promote community safety. Second, it should support local crime prevention efforts and integrate them into community development and health-promoting activities. Third, it should improve services for the victims of crime and those experiencing poor community safety. Overall, respondents called for more 'joining up' of activities at strategic and operational levels. However, they recognised the formidable size of the task of raising awareness and building capacity in order to make this happen.

It was generally agreed that the NHS was not fulfilling its potential. One public health doctor noted:

> We want to tackle inequalities, we want to improve people's lives, and we want to reduce poverty and alleviate its effects. This is broadly the same as regeneration and community safety. So why is there such resistance to working together?

Health service input to local strategic bodies in the community safety arena usually related to specialist services, responding to individual issues (e.g. commissioning of drugs and substance misuse services, participating in mental health teams, and providing regeneration specialists within health promotion). Respondents noted that it was very rare to find a senior individual from the health sector who had, or contributed to, a strategic overview of the complex picture.

Many respondents pointed to the failure of the NHS to participate in local Crime and Disorder partnerships. One local government officer noted: 'It's a miracle if they turn up, and it's an even bigger miracle if they make a contribution.' A

respondent from a non-statutory agency wryly observed: 'If the NHS was clever it would realise that people who walk through the doors of hospitals with injuries caused by street violence or bar-room brawls are using up their precious resources.' For her and many like her, the NHS would feel the benefit of its efforts sooner rather than later, not least in resource terms, if it took its responsibilities for preventing injury to physical and mental health more seriously at both strategic and operational levels.

## STRATEGIC RESPONSIBILITIES

### BUILDING PARTNERSHIPS

As an organisation, the NHS already faces difficulties in performing its traditional role of health care provider. Several respondents made the point that there should be clearer direction from government about the incentives for working together and recognition that small advances require large organisational changes. Indeed, many respondents called for more evidence of joining up activities at the Centre, to 'lead by example'. As one local authority employee commented: 'Get the Department [of Health] to talk to the Home Office; that would be a start.' Others acknowledged that there was joining up at the Centre, but that its impact on local work was limited. Another commented that national initiatives with allocated resources encouraged local action:

> Look at [the national strategy] 'Tackling Drugs Together'. It set out the 'must dos' and came with some money and real progress has been made, because it had to be made, the Government said so ... real money encourages real engagement.

But one respondent noted: 'Nobody spells out what the carrots are, all we see are sticks; it causes resentment.' Lessons should be learned from other relevant attempts to join up action at local levels, including Drug Action Teams and Health Action Zones. And health services would do well to invite community safety agencies to be partners in relevant health initiatives, such as the Local Implementation Groups for Mental Health Services.

Finding capacity to take on additional activities was tough. In addition, it was not always obvious to NHS strategists what the benefits were in taking a bigger role. There was a need for education about the benefits of working closely with others in this field, with resources allocated accordingly. But working more closely entailed risks that policy-makers were reluctant to take. A voluntary sector worker observed: 'People think in institutional ways, they think that it's something the police do, not them ... but it doesn't feel like that if you are in the community.'

NHS managers had to think about services differently and reorientation of those services was needed. However, this would not be easy. As one NHS manager noted:

> Senior managers put the responsibility onto middle management and practitioners to do all the so called 'joining up', yet we don't have the power to really change anything. They do have the power and they should get up off their seats and think outside of their precious little boxes.

The complex relationship between poverty, social exclusion, poor health and high levels of crime in particular localities led many respondents to advocate a greater role for the NHS in regeneration activities, tackling 'upstream' determinants of inequality. The National Strategy for Neighbourhood Renewal was thought to furnish the NHS with considerable opportunities to make a difference locally. Not least, it would enable health service managers to influence some of the decisions not within their power that had direct effects on health. In addition, respondents called for health authorities to integrate targets relating directly to community safety in their Health Improvement Plans, for example action on inequalities. It was suggested that cross-referencing of targets would make it possible to introduce community safety issues into NHS business. Greater NHS contribution to local authority-led Community Strategies was seen as another way in which health targets could become embedded in planning for community safety services and vice versa. As one NHS employee noted: 'We need to start off slowly and build up our efforts ... I look forward to a time when we have community safety targets to meet as part of our mainstream business.'

## INFORMATION SYSTEMS

Respondents recognised that in order to measure achievements in the field, robust and shared systems for measuring performance would have to be developed. Central to the development of relevant strategies was the issue of sharing information across organisations. There were several potential sources of relevant data, but management information systems across sectors were incompatible. For example, A&E departments could make a very useful contribution: simply by recording the number and origin of injuries resulting from violence, they would provide valuable information for police and crime prevention agencies. Young men rarely reported being attacked to the police, therefore police records were often incomplete. Clear ideas about what types of injury were coming from which areas would be beneficial. As one respondent put it:

*We could focus our efforts more effectively, perhaps even know which pubs were producing the highest number of attacks or which families were experiencing domestic violence. If we had this kind of information, we could do much more.*

Close monitoring of the provision of services in response to community safety and crime-related issues would enable the NHS to estimate more accurately the costs of those services as a result of crime. It would demonstrate how NHS involvement in community safety could be beneficial over time. One health authority employee observed: 'We need to look at local areas, where services are, analyse them and understand how our agendas all feed in.' The services of which they spoke fell into two categories: prevention, and treatment and care.

## OPERATIONAL RESPONSIBILITIES

### PREVENTION SERVICES

The NHS was seen to have a clear role in preventing crime and promoting community safety. Respondents described opportunities presented by healthy living centres and other regeneration initiatives to galvanise local action, bringing community members together to identify needs and ways of meeting them, and to initiate action. Several respondents suggested pooling resources to identify issues that had similar causes and to take action on them. For example, one respondent called for life skills programmes with young people that would build confidence, self-esteem, respect for others and basic living skills,

and increase knowledge about sexual health, parenting and how to minimise risk in the misuse of drugs and substances. She hoped that action of this type would meet several objectives at once. Others called for a review of current roles and responsibilities of NHS employees working on the front line; they should be trained in how to promote community safety, for example by assessing the risks faced by individuals, in order to work effectively with those in greatest need: 'Let's be really radical, let's get community nurses, midwives, health visitors in on the community safety work. They know more about what it really means than anyone ever gives them credit for.' The training implications of such changes were seen as extensive.

Protection of NHS staff from harassment, abuse and attack was identified as another area of opportunity. The Department of Health is currently considering this widespread phenomenon and guidelines have been published. However, safety in hospitals and GP surgeries remained a strong concern for many of our interviewees. As one health strategist commented:

*It's about seeing the NHS as part of the community, not something outside of it. Safety issues in hospitals are really very important, whether it is about protecting nurses from being hit or preventing drug dealers getting onto psychiatric wards to get hold of patients' medication. It is all part of the same picture and we should be doing more.*

Several respondents pointed out that vulnerable people in the community, such as drug users, need support, and called for community safety strategists to see them as people with health needs rather than just as criminals: 'We need to remember that drug users are part of our communities. Treating them like the scum of the earth will not in itself make things safer.'

Others observed that young offenders were at risk of depression, experiencing disturbed lives in a culture of violence. They needed support, as did mentally ill people who might be homeless or spend time in public places with nowhere else to go. For the latter, it was more important to find them appropriate support and health services than to criminalise them or pander to those who sought to sweep them off the streets (or as one local authority respondent noted: 'It's not so much sweep them off the street, it's sweep them into another borough, and make them someone else's problem!').

### TREATMENT AND CARE

The NHS as a provider of health services that 'put people back together' and 'pick up the pieces' after they experienced crime was a strong theme in our interviews. Primary care and A&E services were seen to occupy a central role in disseminating information relevant to victims of crime, and referring them on to specialist support services. However, one respondent, a health services researcher observed: 'It's not just about referral, it's about the NHS taking some responsibility and providing services, or at least training staff in how to respond appropriately.' Nurses and doctors were not trained in asking the right questions to be supportive. According to several respondents, GPs resisted asking questions about violence in the home, claiming that it was a matter of privacy and not up to them to make inquiries: 'They [GPs] will ask about the state of your bowels, but they can't bring themselves to ask if you are being beaten at home.' Once again,

training was identified as a means of developing a more integrated response.

Several respondents questioned the legitimacy of codes of confidentiality, claiming that they could endanger people's lives. For example, in cases where women and children were experiencing violence at home, respondents said that it was unacceptable for GPs to resist passing information about individual cases to the police or social services:

> The fact that information should and could be disclosed, well, that's where the NHS becomes unhinged. We know women who live with violent partners are more likely to be attacked during pregnancy. GPs could have a vital role in alerting social services and helping protect the women and their unborn babies.

Several respondents called for a review of current thinking on the question of confidentiality. Most of the discussion on this topic related to GP services, but it was noted that the issues were similar for A&E, sexual health and ward-based services. However, others pointed out that women did not always want information to be passed on to other agencies, or for services to be alerted. They saw such actions as potentially threatening to their well-being, especially when pregnant. Thus, sharing information might deter women from using services. In addition, respondents pointed out that there were extensive problems in making information systems harmonious between, and across, relevant agencies.

### CONCLUSIONS

The research findings presented here suggest a deep frustration at the disjointed relationships between community safety agencies and the NHS in London. There is also considerable enthusiasm about improving that relationship – and 'joining up' – at every level. This should take two forms. First, the NHS should work closely with local authorities and the police, supporting them in strategies for improving community safety and achieving neighbourhood renewal. The benefits for the NHS are clear. Second, the NHS should invite community safety agencies to work closely with it on issues that would benefit from input from a wide range of partners, for example in improving community mental health services. Overall, there is a need to integrate community safety concerns into planning and performance management for the NHS and put them at the very heart of its strategies to reduce inequalities. As one public health specialist said: 'It should be part and parcel of almost everything we do.' Shared targets would drive common agendas and increase the chances of each partner taking its role. Importantly, there needs to be recognition from all quarters that the complexity of the situation will not be addressed through the efforts of any one agency working in isolation. Community safety and health need to be seen holistically: 'We are talking about a whole system re-think,' one health strategist noted. The enthusiasm and commitment of the individuals interviewed for this study could be nurtured and deployed productively to increase professional awareness and stimulate action to improve the safety and health of London's disadvantaged communities.

## ACKNOWLEDGEMENTS

The author would like to thank the respondents who took part in the study. Thanks to Anna Coote and Baljinder Heer for comments on early drafts of this article.

## REFERENCE

Woodhead D. *Community safety and the NHS in London: stakeholder views*. London: King's Fund, 2001.

# DATASCAN

# A rough guide to London's health care web sites

## Valerie Wildridge

*The anarchy of the Internet has allowed the wide proliferation of web sites catering for a wide variety of interest groups. However, this anarchy also makes it difficult to find a specific web site, or sites covering a particular interest.[1]*

Searching the Internet can prove frustrating as well as fruitful. To help navigate some of the web sites devoted to health and health care issues and services in London, this rough guide provides addresses and a short description of the capital's key sites. Many of these have additional links to other London sites (for example, a number of London NHS trusts have now set up their own web sites – go to the London Regional Office site for a list).

### LONDON REGIONAL OFFICE

*www.doh.gov.uk/london*

In May 1998, Frank Dobson announced that 'health services in London will benefit from having a single London Region, instead of being divided between two regions covering the whole of the South-East … '.[2] The London Regional Office (LRO) of the NHS Executive, which officially came into being on 1 April 1999, is responsible for the strategic management of the NHS in London and for health services development and London-wide strategies.

The LRO site follows the same format as that of the NHS Executive's main site and those of the other regional offices. Pages follow in a logical order, taking you from *Welcome* and *What's new*, through the what, who and where of the region, on to *Publications*, and then to major areas of its work within London.

Practical information, such as the map of the region and the number of trusts and primary care groups, is easily found in the section *NHS Executive London*, while the *Directory* lists and provides contact details of all the NHS organisations within the region.

Key reports and briefings by the LRO, and previous Thames Regional Offices,

# Table 1: London health authorities' web addresses

| Health authority | Web address |
| --- | --- |
| Barking and Havering | *www.bhha.org.uk* |
| Barnet, Enfield and Haringey* | *www.ehha.nhs.uk* |
| Bexley, Bromley and Greenwich | *www.bexgreenhealth.nhs.uk* |
| Brent and Harrow | *No web site (at time of writing)* |
| Camden and Islington | *www.cai-ha.nthames.nhs.uk* |
| Croydon | *www.croydon.nhs.uk* |
| Ealing, Hammersmith and Hounslow | *www.ehh-ha.nthames.nhs.uk* |
| East London and The City | *www.elcha.co.uk* |
| Hillingdon | *www.hillingdn-ha.nthames.nhs.uk* |
| Kensington and Chelsea and Westminster | *www.kcwhealth.org.uk* |
| Kingston and Richmond | *www.krha.nhs.uk* |
| Lambeth, Southwark and Lewisham | *www.lslha.nhs.uk* |
| Merton, Sutton and Wandsworth | *www.mswha.nhs.uk* |
| Redbridge and Waltham Forest | *www.rwf-ha.nthames.nhs.uk* |

Note: *Barnet HA and Enfield and Haringey HA merged on 1 April 2001. The web site is still under development and its main content is information from Enfield & Haringey HA.

are available in full text in the *Publications* section – with further reports being found in the various topic areas. The briefings summarising planned improvements in Londoners' health and progress made on those plans, including relevant statistics in the previous quarter, are particularly useful.

The remainder of the site concentrates mainly on the various strategies and projects with which the LRO is involved. These range from *Public Health in London* to *Workforce and Development*. One of particular note is the *Health Strategy for London*, which updates the work of the London Health Commission (see below) and provides links to the London Health Strategy document,[3] other meeting reports, rapid reviews and newsletters. These pages are currently being reconfigured and should be available shortly at *www.londonshealth.gov.uk*

The LRO web site is an important start for anyone looking at London health policy.

## LONDON HEALTH AUTHORITIES

Space does not permit a review of all the London health authority or, especially, hospital sites. Some are still under development, and the quality of those available can be variable. Generally, these sites tend to cover the same types of information: what service provision there is within the authority; contacts for those services; and downloadable copies of annual reports, public health annual reports and Health Improvement Programmes. Table 1 gives web addresses for health authorities.

## LONDON HEALTH COMMISSION

*www.london.gov.uk/mayor/health_commission/ health_index.htm*

The London Health Commission was established in 2000 to advise the Mayor of London on health-related issues. It is taking forward plans proposed in the London Health Strategy[4] to improve health and reduce inequalities across London. The Commission consists of around 40 members from different sectors and has six sponsors: the Greater London Authority, the LRO, the King's Fund, the Association of London Government, the Government Office for London, and the Social Services Inspectorate for London. For more background information on the Commission, visit

*www.london.gov.uk/mayor/health_commission/ oct12agenda/papers/hlthoct12item3.pdf*

The site includes details of what the London Health Commission is and who its members are. Thereafter, the main focus of the site is the meetings of the Commission, with dates, agendas and minutes provided. The minutes include links to full text reports that have been written for the Commission.

The Commission's pages keep you in touch at all times with the mayor's web site and those of the Greater London Authority, both starting at *www.london. gov.uk*

The site holds a wealth of information of relevance to improving Londoners' health and, while it does not have a search facility, it is certainly worthwhile visiting.

## VIRTUALL, THE LONDON MENTAL HEALTH LEARNING PARTNERSHIP

*www.virtuall.org*

Virtuall is 'a partnership connecting health, social care, justice, service users, carers and non-statutory organisations to progress the Strategy for Mental Health in London'.[5] It aims to establish good practice in mental health across London, to support staff in improving mental health care across sectors, e.g. health, housing, police, and to be involved in key changes in the health and social care fields.

The Virtuall site holds a number of articles, unpublished reports and links that are of relevance to anyone working with people with mental health problems. There is a useful alerting service, whereby you can register to receive e-mails of newly added content of particular interest to you. The site also includes details of events and training courses.

## LONDON AMBULANCE SERVICE

*www.lond-amb.sthames.nhs.uk*

The London Ambulance Service (LAS) works over the whole of Greater London, with 70 ambulance stations providing cover to the 7 million people in the capital at any one time. It responds to approximately 1500 accident and emergency calls per day. For more detailed information, visit

*www.lond-amb.sthames.nhs.uk/http.dir/ service/ser_menu.html*

Those interested in the work of the LAS should find all they need to know on this site, including a detailed description of its service (see above for the specific page), its performance review and its service plan. The *Links* page will take you to other ambulance services around the country.

## LONDON HEALTH OBSERVATORY

*www.lho.org.uk*

One of the eight public health observatories covering each NHS region, the London Health Observatory (LHO) was established to fulfil an objective in the White Paper *Saving Lives: Our Healthier Nation*.[6] The LHO aims to collate information and datasets on health in London, and to analyse and disseminate this information to help those working and lobbying for Londoners' health. Further information on their role can be found at

*www.lho.org.uk/lho/pdf/LHO.pdf*

This is a goldmine of information and excellently put together, though it is still under development and it can take a little time to read the tickertape on the home page, which informs you of new additions to the site. Grouped under *Determinants of Health*, *Lifestyle and behaviour*, *Disease groups* and *Population groups*, it looks at health in London from various perspectives, giving almost all the 32 topics listed a descriptive overview, access to some local data where possible, and links to relevant experts, organisations and resources. Its *Publications* page includes not only their own reports but those of other key London health organisations, such as the Health of Londoners Project and the King's Fund, with links to full text where possible. A comprehensive index and a simple search facility adds to the accessibility of the information on this site.

## HEALTH OF LONDONERS PROJECT

*www.elcha.co.uk/holp*

The Health of Londoners Project (HoLP) was set up in early 1995 with funding from the two Thames Regional Health Authorities and the London Implementation Group. It provides a centre for London-wide health information and analysis, looking at data at health or local authority level, but also with some ward-level analyses. It carries out focused project work, for example the effect of transport issues on health, and works closely with other London agencies.

The HoLP web site carries details of its current work and publications, most of which are available in full text. One useful aspect of the site is a listing of the Greater London health authorities and the London boroughs that fall within each HA, with links to contact details and web sites where available. A word of caution though: at the time of writing, these links had not been updated since November 2000 and research for this article showed more London HAs now have web sites (see Table 1).

## KING'S FUND

*www.kingsfund.org.uk*

Founded over 100 years ago, the King's Fund is an independent health care charity, whose main focus is working to improve the health of Londoners by making change happen in health and social care. This is done by carrying out research, through development work, and by developing people and encouraging new ideas.

With a new web manager in post, the site is set to improve on its already informative pages and to be quicker and easier to search. Clicking on *What we do* on the *Home* page takes you to the various teams and groups within the Fund and to the breadth of projects with which they are involved. Contact details are given and, where possible, full text access to documentation supporting the projects, as well as evaluative and research reports.

In August 2001, the Fund launched a virtual e-bookshop, *www.kingsfundbook shop.org.uk*, offering access to a good proportion of the stock held on health and social care management and enabling visitors to order online.

Finally, for anyone wanting to search the Internet for health policy information but not quite sure where to start, the excellent *Links* page is a must. It will take you not only to the sites mentioned in this article, but also to a vast array of health service engines and government, academic and voluntary agencies sites involved in health policy, most with a one-line description.

## IMAGINE LONDON

*www.imaginelondon.org.uk*

Set up in 1998 by the King's Fund, Imagine London is a five-year programme to develop and reflect young people's views, feelings and visions for the future health of London through digital diaries and conference reports. It targets issues the young people have raised themselves, such as air quality, traffic and lifestyle.

## LONDON HEALTH EMERGENCY

*http://freespace.virgin.net/health.emergency/ home.htm*

London Health Emergency (LHE) describes itself as 'the country's biggest and longest-running pressure group in defence of the NHS'.[7] It provides independent research, monitoring and information on all aspects of health care in London. It has been actively involved in campaigns to prevent hospital closures within London, and works with other local organisations with an interest in health care issues.

Quite compact, this site has a welcoming feel to it, with easy-to-use pages asking you to *join us* or send in *enquiries*. Although the number of pages is limited, what is there is all relevant. The *home* page has a description of the research and campaigning with which the LHE is involved, and takes you to its latest newsletter. In addition, it helps to produce newsletters for some UNISON branches, and samples of these are also included. The LHE researches issues for trade unions and campaigners, and a number of the subsequent reports can be found in the *research documents* (unfortunately not all the links appeared to be working as I was testing them). The *links* page lists mainly trade union organisations and campaigning groups.

## LONDON VOLUNTARY SERVICE COUNCIL

*www.lvsc.org.uk*

The London Voluntary Service Council (LVSC) aims to provide services that strengthen London's voluntary organisations, and speaks with a strong voice on policy issues that affect Londoners.

This site will give you an overview of the work of the LVSC, a description of the subject stock held in its library, details of its publications, and funding and contact details. It does not contain in-depth information or links to full text documents. These can be found at a project in which it is taking the lead – Action Link London.

## ACTION LINK LONDON

*www.actionlink.org.uk*

The aim of Action Link London is to bring together information on the capital's voluntary sector activities and make this information more accessible. Information found there should include: a guide to the voluntary sector in London; jobs and training courses; and a knowledge library for the voluntary sector.

At the time of writing, Action Link was undergoing final testing, which might account for its tardiness. Where there was information available, in the *News* and *Events* sections, for example, it was certainly current. The *Resources* section includes relevant documents (though the links don't always work) and sites for those interested in or working with the voluntary sector.

Not immediately obvious are two sections below the *Organisations* banner. *Action Link Direct* lists London voluntary groups and can be searched according to types of organisations, the target groups with which they work, and the geographical area they serve and work in. Also under *Organisations* is *Action Link Guides*, a series of guides aimed at voluntary organisations and covering topics such as information technology, personnel and training. A useful site for exploring what the voluntary sector is doing in London, possibly for learning from each other when their *Discussion* pages get going; and for finding partners in areas of similar interest.

## LONDONHEALTH

*www.londonhealth.co.uk*

LondonHealth is a site aimed at the general public, offering a free, fully searchable database of health-related practitioners, professionals, organisations, information sources, etc., in the Greater London area. It states that its mission is

to be 'London's one-stop Internet health and fitness information provider'.[8]

A useful site for those new to London, it provides information on how to locate a doctor, dentist or chemist in a given postcode area, and lists details of specific subject organisations; however, if using the contact details, do check the currency of the information, some of which does not appear to have been updated recently.

## LONDON MEDICINE

*www.londonmedicine.org.uk*

London Medicine is a non-profit-making organisation that aims to increase awareness of London's medical expertise and to encourage clinical, academic and commercial partnerships between London and the rest of the world.

A wide variety of information is contained within this site as it aims to cater for a diverse community. Included on the site are *50 facts about London Medicine*, which contains facts and figures on medical treatment, education and research, and other areas. However, do check the accuracy of the statistics quoted as at the foot of the page a 1997 disclaimer is given; this is true of several of their pages, most noticeably their list of useful organisations for supplies – 0171/0181 numbers have not been updated. Still, quite a useful site for giving an overview of medical treatment in the capital, but with a more commercial slant.

## RACE ON THE AGENDA

*www.rota.org.uk*

Race On The Agenda (ROTA) is a policy development information and research service for the black voluntary sector in

London, working towards the elimination of discrimination and to promote both equality of opportunity and best practice.

On entering the site, its bold black background and red print looks exciting. Unfortunately, it does not contain a great deal of information nor does it give you an indication of currency. It states that its *Links* are forthcoming – but when? What it does hold is its newsletter (not updated since 1998) and a couple of briefing papers. However, I understand that the site is currently being developed, so one to keep any eye on if you are particularly focusing on black issues in London.

## BLACK REGENERATION FORUM

*www.cemvo.org.uk/brf/brf.htm*

The Black Regeneration Forum is a partnership organisation aiming to bring together local and regional networks of black-led organisations.

Held on the Ethnic Minority Foundation (EMF) and the Council of Ethnic Minority Voluntary Sector Organisations (CEMVO) web site, this page outlines the aims and objectives of the Forum, its partners, and links to three full text documents: social exclusion and neighbourhood renewal; connecting communities; and the Urban White Paper. Like ROTA, not a great deal of information, but a starting point.

## LONDON 21

*www.london21.org*

London 21's mission is 'to assist London's communities and all those engaged in personal and community-based action for sustainability in the Greater London area to find mutual support and link their work with the actions of others who have similar goals'.[9]

The site includes a *Directory* of over 1000 organisations working towards sustainability in London. The *Directory* can be searched either by subject, e.g. *Community Focus, Health and Home, Policy, Politics and Planning*, or by organisation name or keyword. A *Conferencing* section enables you to join discussions or start your own conference space. There is also a *Public Events Database*, though there didn't appear to be many events listed. I particularly liked this site for its clear messages about what each section is for and how to use it. It is a very friendly and useful site for those interested in sustainability in London.

## LONDON LIVE

*www.bbc.co.uk/londonlive*

Part of the BBC's site, and as the name implies, it focuses on news and entertainment in London. The reason for including it here is its section *United Colours of London*, which is a guide to some of the cultures in the capital. Organised by cultural group, each section contains a page on health care leading to useful local organisations that cater to the particular ethnic group.

## REFERENCES

1 Tyrell S. *Using the Internet in healthcare*. Abingdon: Radcliffe Medical Press, 1999.
2 Department of Health. *Frank Dobson announces new London-wide health region: single London Regional Office to be created on 1st April 1999*. Press release 98/19, 18 May 1998.
3 London Health Strategy Steering Group. *The London health strategy: outline strategic framework: March 2000*. London: NHS Executive, 2000.
4 *Ibid*.
5 Virtuall. *More about us. http://www.virtuall. org/more_about.html*

6 Department of Health. *Saving lives: our healthier nation.* London: Stationery Office, 1999.

7 London Health Emergency. *Pressure group.* *http://freespace.virgin.net/health.emergency/ home.htm*

8 LondonHealth. *Mission statement.* *http:// www. londonhealth.co.uk*

9 London 21. *Mission statement.* *http:// www.london21.org*